From the pages of
Handbook for Human Potential

"Your body has been waiting patiently,
welcome home to your body wisdom."
— Chandra Zas

"Unlearn performance as identity and relearn movement as medicine."
— Dr. Nikia Evans

"Breath is your access point to better sleep."
— Keaton Lynn

"When Qi is moving freely, your
mind and body will feel more in the flow."
— Dr. Erika Siegel

"Prevention is key. Impact your health through diet and lifestyle."
— Dr. Erin Frances Sharman

"You can have amazing nutritional density
in your blood, and your cells are starving."
— Julie North

"Resilience isn't just enduring hardship — it's thriving through it."
— Seth Eliot

"Stop chasing who you think you should be
and start living as who you are."
— Diana Elizabeth

"It's easier to move through life when you're aligned with love."
— Teresa Rodriguez

"We must re-wild as a human society, and that starts with you."
— Mac Murphy

"It doesn't matter how clean you eat if you are stressed."
— Chandra Zas

"Trauma creates a long-term impact on your well-being."
— Jim Pehkonen

"Trauma starts when your breath stops."
— Yotam Tamari

"Psychedelics help the brain rewire itself
and potentially regain lost function."
— Dr. Burton J. Tabaac

"Ketamine is a life-changing and life-saving medicine."
— Greg Jones

"Erotic energy is a potent force that makes the world go round."
— Usha Rose

"It is not true that at any point in life it's too late to begin."
— Dr. Maria Cristina

"Your current life is only one part of your soul journey."
— Britta Jo

"Living while dying is a magnificent,
triumphant expression of being human."
— Patricia Moir Pollman

HANDBOOK FOR HUMAN POTENTIAL

HANDBOOK
for
HUMAN POTENTIAL

An accessible guide to personal growth

Foreword by Jeffrey J. Kripal

Compiled and edited by Chandra Zas

Cover design: Chandra Zas
Interior design: SHR Book Design

To My Big Love – you know who you are –
this book exists because of your support.
Thank you for always having my back.

To My Little Love – I love you. Even when... and
always.

To each author who said yes to this book's
vision – thank you for contributing your
wisdom, energy, and love.

To My Dear Mother – Thank you for teaching
me to love reading and writing.

To You, Dear Reader – Thank you for being
here and doing "the work."

How to use this book

The chapters in this book, contain tools and wisdom for you to take into your mind, body, heart, and your life.

I encourage you to scan the table of contents with an unfocused gaze and see if you are drawn to a particular chapter. Trust that intuitive pull – it often reveals what your journey needs most right now. Or go for the chapter that you want to, or read it in order. Your choice.

The beauty of this handbook is that it's designed for your unique path. You might start with Part Two if your body is calling for attention or jump to Part Four if healing trauma feels most urgent. Perhaps Part Three's inner tools resonate, or Part Five's deeper territories call to you. Part One offers a welcoming home to access into your body wisdom – a great place to start.

Read, reflect, and implement at your own pace. Turn the page and begin.

Chandra Zas
Book momma

Contents

Foreword   xi

Introduction   1

Part One: Welcome

0 | Come Home to Your Body Wisdom   7
    Chandra Zas

Part Two: Functional Body Care

1 | Minimum Effective Dose: A Return to Holistic Movement   27
    Dr. Nikia Evans

2 | Breath and Sleep: The Missing Links to Your Foundation   41
    Keaton Lynn

3 | The Nuts and Bolts of Chinese Medicine   57
    Dr. Erika Siegel

4 | Naturopathic Medicine from Womb to Wisdom Years   71
    Dr. Erin Frances Sharman

5 | The Core Fix for Starving Cells: Trace Minerals and Cell Salts   85
    Julie North

Part Three: Inner Tools

6 | Frameworks for Facing Hard Times   103
    Seth Eliot

7 | Discovering Your Human Design: Where It All Begins   121
    Diana Elizabeth

8 | Live in the Frequency of Love   143
    Teresa Rodriguez

9 | Right Relation through Elemental Embodiment   157
    Mac Murphy

10 | Mood Before Food   175
    Chandra Zas

Part Four: Brain Changers for Healing

11 | Heal Deep Trauma to Create an Alive Life   195
    Jim Pehkonen

12 | Minimize the Lasting Impact of Pain and Suffering with   209
Therapeutic Breathing
    Yotam Tamari

13 | Brain Healing with Psychedelics   227
    Dr. Burton J. Tabaac

14 | Ketamine for Mental Health   243
    Greg Jones

Part Five: Beyond the Daily Grind

15 | Sexually Empowered and Erotically Embodied   267
    Usha Rose

16 | Gaining Vitality While Reimagining Aging   285
    Dr. Maria Cristina

17 | Create a Soul-Led Life   295
    Britta Jo

18 | The Sacred Exit: The Journey of Sacred Passages   311
    Patricia Moir Pollman

Epilogue: Life Design 101   325

Acknowledgments   331

Foreword

The Same Love That Moves the Stars

Dr. Jeffrey J. Kripal

Let me begin at the end. The exit. It has struck me many times over the years that the midwestern American culture from which I emerged tends to pathologize death. Basically, it makes death something bad. Death, or so it seems, is always someone's fault. It is a matter of responsibility. He drank too much. She ate too much. They did not see a doctor. And so on. I often think to myself, "But why can't we just let people die? Is not death the natural ending of an organic life?"

What these chapters accomplish is mostly before such an ending, but they are very much about that same organic nature—about those molecules, emotions, and energies, about what we are. On one level, I suppose, they can be read as exhortations to do this or that, or not do this or that. On another deeper level, though, they are not about any of those things. They are not about that guilt or badness. Quite the opposite: they are about a fundamental goodness. They are about the Earth, sleep, balance, breath, relationship, diet, self, soul, emotion, love, sexuality, aging, psychedelic molecules, and trauma. They are about life as wholeness.

Language matters. One hears sometimes about "embodiment" or "having" a body. But there is an implied dualism in such words. Maybe that is what grammar does—split us. But not here. We do not just "have" bodies here. We are those bodies, which are so similar and yet also so very different. These chapters give us very practical ways to be those bodies.

I have this bookmark on my desk. It quotes the paleontologist, priest, and writer Teilhard de Chardin about how love is the same force that moves the stars. I think such a statement is usually read metaphorically (or maybe it is a distant reference to Dante), but the writer almost certainly meant it more literally. We, after all, are cosmic and evolutionary in our very natures. The bookmark is not engaging in metaphors. It is speaking that truth, if we can hear it.

These authors show us something similar—we are the evolving universe becoming aware of itself. If that is not human potential, I do not know what human potential is. These chapters also represent a new generation of authors, activists, bodyworkers, and healers. May we be changed accordingly. May we hear and be changed.

Jeffrey J. Kripal
J. Newton Rayzor Professor of
Philosophy and Religious Thought
August 2025

Introduction

I hold hope for new, aligned, systems to arise both personally and collectively. I have great frustration with our current medical, food, and insurance systems because they are incentivized for profit rather than health and wellbeing. I have organized this handbook because I know there are real remedies for the mental, emotional, physical, and spiritual struggles that plague many of us.

For you, who are on the path of growth and self-development, this handbook is created to accompany you on your journey of both overcoming your struggles and embracing your potential. Each person's greatest potential is unique yet shares common patterns that can guide us all.

What you hold in your hands is a compilation of lived experience from devoted practitioners, bodyworkers, guides, healers, mediums, nurses, and doctors across diverse fields – from physical to mental and emotional to spiritual – all united by a single purpose: to help you unlock what you are truly capable of when you have the tools you need.

Many of you are here to grow, called to transmute intergenerational pains and patterns, moved to consciously evolve, usher in new systems, heal, and expand. In my own multi-decade journey of overcoming personal pains and sufferings, I have experienced hundreds of different modalities, perspectives, teachers, healers, and masters – gaining reverence for the vast number of paths that twist and turn but ultimately lead to relieving suffering and increasing human potential.

There is no magic pill, yet there is much you can do in your everyday life that will accumulate to create what you desire.

I think of this journey as being like a puzzle with many pieces or even a recipe with a basic set of ingredients that can be swapped out and upgraded. There are many pieces to each of our puzzles; sometimes there is a piece that doesn't fit yet, because there are other pieces that need to connect into place first.

My aim in creating this book is to give you optional pieces for your puzzle, upgraded ingredients for your personal recipe – ones that benefit both you personally as well as raise our collective wellbeing.

The journey through five parts

The chapters ahead are organized to support your growth from foundation to transformation, structured in five distinct yet interconnected parts:

Part One: Come Home to Your Body Wisdom – reconnecting with your internal guidance system. This chapter offers practical pathways for tuning back into your body's wisdom and authentic desire.

Part Two: Functional Body Care focuses on the physical foundation of your wellbeing. Here you'll discover holistic approaches to movement, the wisdom of Chinese and naturopathic medicine, the critical importance of breath and sleep, and how trace minerals and cell salts can address cellular starvation. These chapters provide the embodied foundation that supports all other growth.

Part Three: Inner Tools offers frameworks and practices for consciousness work. You'll explore approaches for facing hard times, discover your unique Human Design blueprint, learn to live in the frequency of love, and understand elemental embodiment. These tools help you navigate life's challenges from a place of inner resourcefulness.

Part Four: Brain Changers for Healing examines cutting-edge approaches to healing trauma and optimizing mental health. From therapeutic breathing and deep trauma work to the emerging field of psychedelic medicine and ketamine therapy, these chapters address the profound healing possible when we work directly with the brain and nervous system.

Part Five: Beyond the Daily Grind ventures into the territories that give life its deepest meaning – sexuality and embodiment, creating a soul-led life, reimagining aging with vitality, and approaching death as a sacred transition. These chapters invite you into the fullest expression of human potential.

Each teacher brings their unique knowledge and lived experience, offering practical tools to help you navigate your path with greater awareness, vitality, and purpose. Whether you're seeking physical wellness, emotional balance, deeper relationships, or expanded consciousness, you'll find guidance from authors who have dedicated their lives to these transformative practices.

Part One

Welcome

0

Come Home to Your Body Wisdom

Chandra Zas

I was on autopilot, seeking a little distraction from lack of sleep and the radical adjustment of parenthood. "I'm just checking this one thing," I'd tell myself as my daughter nestled in my arms. "She's too young to notice." "I can multitask." But my body knew better. There was a hollow feeling in my chest, a disconnection I couldn't ignore. When I stopped distracting myself and started listening to what my body was telling me, I realized I was stealing presence – from her, and from myself.

This seemingly small moment became a profound turning point. It wasn't just about putting my phone down; it was about recognizing a pattern of disconnection that had been quietly running my life. It was about waking up to the subtle ways I was choosing distraction over presence, numbness over feeling, and external noise over my own inner wisdom. It was a pivotal moment where I understood that my body was speaking to me, and that I had the choice to listen.

That moment of awareness changed both my relationship to my phone and my capacity to listen to my body's signals. It was one of the defining moments in my journey toward functional embodiment. **Functional embodiment is beyond noticing sensations; it is using body cues, body signals, and body wisdom as an internal guidance system to make choices that create well-being.**

In our current world of endless information and quick-fix solutions, it's easy to lose touch with our body's wisdom. It is easy to mindlessly scroll or emotionally snack. These are normal responses to modern culture and common symptoms of living disconnected from our body wisdom. We are conditioned to look outside of ourselves for answers, to follow the latest trends, and to ignore the subtle signals of our own bodies. Many of us are taught to override our hunger cues with diet plans, to avoid our emotions with distractions, and to push down our pains with alcohol. But this way of living comes at a cost. It leaves us feeling disconnected, unfulfilled, and out of sync with our own bodies and lives.

Pathways: Welcome home to your body wisdom

The pathway to embodiment is a path where you pull the strings for your own well-being. You know your own algorithm. It is a way of living in which you make tuned-in choices, according to your internal guidance system, from food and screen time consumption to daily life decisions.

If you're reading this, something inside you is already stirring toward change. Perhaps you've felt that same hollow disconnection I experienced, or maybe you feel the call to connect with your body's wisdom. Whatever brought you here, I want to acknowledge the courage it takes to look inward and the intelligence of your inner guidance that led you to this moment. This chapter offers you five pathways back home to your functional embodiment. These aren't mystical concepts but practical tools you can use immediately to create clarity, calm, and connection in your body, mind, and life. My wish for you is that you'll step into your functional embodiment by honoring your body wisdom, and trusting the internal guidance system that's been within you all along.

Pathway 1: Honor your body's signals and feedback

Start with the foundation – our body's innate wisdom. Our body is constantly communicating through cues, signals, and messages. From our cellular needs to our gut instincts, plus messages from our intuition and even our microbes, we each have an internal feedback system that can guide everything from screen and food choices to life decisions.

Many of us learned to override these signals early in life. "Finish your plate." "Sit still." "Don't be so sensitive." These well-meaning instructions taught us to ignore our body's feedback in favor of external rules. We learned to value external validation over our own internal knowing. We were praised for being "good" and for following the rules, even when it meant ignoring our own cues, signals, and body wisdom. This conditioning runs deep; it can take time and practice to unlearn these old patterns and to start trusting our own bodies again.

The practice:

Start with simple body awareness around food and water.

Notice when you drink treated restaurant water – does your mouth constrict and say no? Have you experienced drinking fresh spring water and felt your body's visceral yes instinct? This is a simple but profound way to start listening to your body's feedback. Pay attention to the subtle sensations in your mouth and throat. Does the water feel hydrating and nourishing, or does it feel harsh and hard to swallow? Your body knows the difference, and it will tell you if you are willing to listen.

Observe when you eat, are you choosing salads because you think they're healthy, or because your body's instinct is signaling yes? Are you regularly binging on highly processed foods knowing you will feel off after? Are you forcing "healthy" foods down while ignoring your body's instinctual feedback?

My story:

When I was pregnant, my midwife insisted I needed iron supplements. My body said no – loudly. I fought myself for months, forcing down pills that did not sit well. Genetic testing later revealed my body has a genetic inability to process that type of iron. My body knew something my mind and my midwife didn't. This experience was a powerful reminder that my body is not a machine to be fixed or controlled. It is a living, breathing organism with its own intelligence and wisdom. It is my potential ally or my cage; it is always communicating with me. If I want it to be my ally then my duty is to listen, to trust, and to honor the messages it sends me.

I use my body for guidance with most choices including social events, work decisions, parenting, screen time, and food. I tune into my body's yes/no instinct before as well as how my body responds to what I take in – physically, mentally, and emotionally.

Your turn:

Start paying attention to your body's instinctual yes/no signals. When your body says, "No, do not drink this water, eat this food, take this pill" – honor your instinct. When you think about hanging out with a friend and your energy contracts, consider changing your plans. Your body's wisdom has been refined over millions of years of evolution. Trust it.

Take a moment to appreciate that you're already invested in this journey simply by reading these words. Your body has been waiting patiently for you to return to this conversation. Welcome home to your own inner wisdom.

Pathway 2: Befriend your uncomfortable emotions

As you bring your awareness to your body's signals, you're already practicing embodiment. Notice how it feels to even consider trusting your internal guidance again. Now that you're tuning into your body's signals, you'll likely notice uncomfortable emotions arising. This is where most people reach for distractions like scrolling, snacking, and drinking. But these quick fixes create more problems than they solve.

At the root of human motivation is emotion: we're driven to feel good and avoid feeling bad. Our brains naturally seek pleasure, avoid pain, and seek efficiency. So, it's completely normal to want to escape uncomfortable emotions. But this avoidance is costly.

My story:

I went through a painful breakup and felt depression creeping in. My therapist offered me a remedy that worked: "Feel as long and as hard as you can." After our session, I sat in my car and let a wave of grief arise. I decided to be brave and allow myself to feel it fully. I cried hard for a few minutes and then felt much lighter, even refreshed.

Use your mind's conscious choice to overcome your brain's tendency to avoid emotional pain and to instead befriend your feelings. You will feel far better once you get the hang of it.

The car analogy tool:

Imagine you're driving a car, and your emotions are your passengers. Maybe overwhelm and fear are in the back seat; perhaps anger is riding shotgun. Instead of trying to kick them out of the car, treat them like friends. Talk to them, ask questions, get curious about what they need. You stay the driver – you hold the wheel and make decisions – but you create a connected, curious relationship with all your passengers.

This analogy is so useful because it shifts the way you relate to your emotions. Instead of seeing them as enemies to be vanquished, you can see them as messengers to be heard. Your emotions are not the problem; they are the symptom. They are pointing you to something that needs your attention. When you practice listening to your emotions with curiosity and compassion, you won't *need* emotional distractions like snacking or scrolling.

Depression has been a passenger in my car many times. I've learned that when depression shows up, it's usually because I'm avoiding an uncomfortable emotion. If I ignore depression, it takes control of my car. If I get curious and lean in, allowing my uncomfortable emotions space, then my depression is lifted.

The numbing spectrum:

Beyond scrolling and snacking, many people have learned to use alcohol as a legal emotional numbing tool. The evening glass of wine to "take the edge off," the weekend drinks to "decompress," the social drinking to feel more comfortable – alcohol is culturally normalized as a coping mechanism. Alcohol temporarily dampens our nervous system, creating the illusion of relief while actually preventing us from processing the emotions that need our attention – often leaving residues of anxiety, depression, and inflammation.

The practice:

When you feel the urge to scroll, snack, or drink, pause and ask: "Am I doing this to avoid an emotion?" See what happens to your body if you instead lean in and feel that emotion. Put your hand on your chest. Take a few breaths. Get curious about its message. This is uncomfortable in the moment but creates long-term emotional well-being.

I've witnessed a renaissance in people exploring microdosing and plant medicines as alternatives to traditional numbing. Unlike alcohol and SSRIs, which tend to suppress feelings, plant medicines can increase the capacity to feel, connect, and process emotions. When used with intention and proper guidance, they can help access and make peace at the root causes of patterns rather than attempting to avoid emotional pains.

The key distinction is this: are you using something to avoid feeling, or to make peace with your emotions? Are you seeking to numb out, or to connect? Alcohol typically serves the former, while conscious plant medicine work serves the latter. Both require honest self-reflection about your intentions.

Whether you choose to explore plant medicines or not, the fundamental practice remains the same: developing the capacity to be present with your emotions without immediately reaching for something to change how you feel. This is the pathway to genuine emotional freedom – not the temporary relief of numbing, but the lasting peace that comes from befriending all parts of your emotional landscape.

Pathway 3: Mindfully consume

As you embody and befriend your emotions, you'll naturally gain mindfulness of what you're consuming – mentally and physically. Mindfulness naturally leads to making choices from your body wisdom that lead to well-being.

Think of your mind like a supercomputer – what you think affects your body: how you feel and what you do. Marketers know your algorithm; it is to your advantage to know your algorithm too. "I deserve a snack" creates desire for a snack. "I can't have just one" leads to compulsive eating. Marketers know the messaging that creates feelings like fear, scarcity, desire, and urgency to influence your behavior.

The digital detox:

Just as you've hopefully learned to read nutrition labels on food, you need to become conscious of the "nutrition" of your mental and emotional consumption. Your media information and screen time consumption are processed through your brain, body, and nervous system, which affects not only how you immediately feel and behave but also how you digest and sleep.

I notice that the news invokes fear and stress, while some podcasts invoke curiosity and motivation. The key is noticing the effects and choosing intentionally.

The dopamine trap:

Your devices are designed to hijack your dopamine system – the same system that governs addiction. Every notification, like, and scroll triggers a small hit of dopamine, keeping you coming back for more. This creates a cycle that leaves you mindlessly scrolling and missing the simple pleasures of life, like a sunset, a smile, or a cup of tea.

Breaking free from this cycle requires conscious choice about what you allow into your mental space. It means curating your consumption based on how you want to feel rather than just consuming whatever is put in front of you. It means deciding ahead of time and using your inner tools to follow through on your decision.

The practice:

Use your awareness to choose ahead of time how you want to feel. Ask yourself:

- How does scrolling versus watching a sunset make me feel?
- How does snacking versus going for a walk affect my energy?
- **How do I want to feel?**

From temporary to long-term:

Your brain evolved to seek immediate pleasure, but connecting to your body's feedback switches your choices from costly instant gratification to long-term well-being.

Before making choices, ask: "How do I want to feel in two hours? Tomorrow morning? Ten years from now?"

Digital practices:

Creating intentional practices with technology is essential for your embodiment. This might mean phone-free meals, no screens for the first hour of your day, turning off many of your notifications, or designated times for checking messages. These don't need to be rules to follow rigidly but embodied experiments in reclaiming your attention, presence, and well-being.

I've found that the quality of my morning sets the tone for my entire day. When I start with checking my phone, I'm less present and feel more scattered for the day. When I start my day with a warm cup of tea, snuggles with my dog, and enjoying the view out my window, I remain grounded in my body throughout the day.

Your thoughts are the code to your supercomputer

Paying attention to your thoughts will help you get to know your own algorithm and choose the code to your mind's supercomputer. Thoughts containing words like 'have to,' 'should,' 'always,' 'never,' 'can't,' 'supposed,' 'everyone,' and 'no one' – are words that I recommend paying attention to by flagging and questioning them.

Questioning your code:
Start flagging and questioning thoughts containing "have to" or "should" – these often signal inherited conditioning rather than authentic choice.

My example:
The thought "I have to pay my parking ticket" creates pressure – and isn't even true. I could not pay it, get fined, have my license revoked. That's an option. Instead, realizing "I want to keep my license, so part of me wants to pay this ticket" has connection, truth, and motivation.

The practice:
Create an inner alliance with your thinking. Notice how different thoughts affect your body; then, mindfully choose thoughts that align with how you want to feel and behave. This is not about positive thinking or ignoring reality. It is about recognizing that you have a choice in how you think and interact with the world around you. This is embodied mindfulness in action. Get to know your algorithm, your mind's supercomputer, and make choices that are connected to your body wisdom.

Pathway 4: Clarify your expectations and make requests

Once you begin to practice mindful screentime and intentional thinking, you'll likely notice how many unconscious expectations are running in the background of your mind. These hidden expectations often drive emotional reactions more than the actual events themselves.

Nothing creates emotional upset like unmet expectations. Yet how many of your expectations are clear and communicated? Getting clear within yourself and communicating your expectations and requests to others will relieve disconnect, frustration, and stress.

The invisible rulebook:

Most people carry around an invisible rulebook about how people "should" behave – rules inherited from families, culture, and past experiences. These unconscious expectations create friction when reality doesn't match the internal script.

My story:

I grew up believing men should put the toilet seat down. My partner didn't grow up with this idea. When I asked him to put it down, he asked me to put it up. I realized I could either accept this difference or keep feeling irritated. I chose to change my expectation.

The cost of unconscious expectations:

When you hold unconscious expectations, you're essentially demanding that reality be different than it is. This creates a state of resistance and disconnect. You waste enormous amounts of emotional energy being frustrated by things that are simply part of the human experience – people being imperfect, differences, plans changing, life's duality.

Expectations vs. requests:

Learning to distinguish between expectations and requests has been life-changing for me. I can request that people are on time without expecting it. I can request that my partner puts down the lid without expecting it. This shift allows me to communicate my requests clearly while staying emotionally embodied and accepting when they're not met.

Common unconscious expectations:

- "Friends should call on my birthday."

- "People should be on time."

- "Kids should behave."

- "People shouldn't lie, cheat, or steal."

The truth is: friends don't always call, people are sometimes late, kids do get dysregulated – people do lie, cheat, and steal. Thinking they "should not" creates disconnect.

The practice of clear requests:

This doesn't mean becoming passive or accepting harmful behavior. It means accepting reality as it is so you can respond from clarity rather than reactivity. Put your hand on your heart, look inward for what it is you want – not because you think they should but because the grounded present version of you *wants*. When I accept that my friend is often late, I can create systems that work for both of us rather than feeling personally wounded by their lateness.

Communicating requests:

Once you're clear about your expectations, you can communicate your requests without attachment to the outcome. "I'd like to make a request that we have phone-free dinners" is different from "You have to put your phone away during dinner." The first invites collaboration; the second creates disconnect.

The practice:

Notice where you're thinking or saying people "should" or "shouldn't" do something. Get curious about your expectations. Sometimes awareness alone is relieving. Other times, tuning into your body wisdom, getting internally clear on your want, and having a vulnerable conversation about your requests can create important connection and clarity.

Becoming clear about your expectations creates emotional spaciousness, which reduces your need to cope through snacking, scrolling, or drinking.

Pathway 5: Connect with your inner characters

You've begun your journey of reconnection by getting this far in my chapter. I am glad you are here investing your time and attention. Each pathway has been an invitation back home to your body wisdom. To use your inner guidance system requires your presence and attention. Beyond your brain's supercomputer thinking and your body wisdom, you have inner characters or parts of who you are, that are worthy of getting to know.

The embodied self:

You are not one unified self but a collection of different parts, each with their own needs, desires, and perspectives. The part of you that wants to eat healthy is different from the part that craves comfort food. The part that wants to be productive is different from the part that needs rest. When these parts are in conflict and you're unconscious of them, you feel fragmented, exhausted, and at war with yourself.

Common inner parts:

While everyone's inner landscape is unique, there are some common characters that many people recognize:

- The inner child: Holds your wonder, creativity, and need for play, but also your wounds and unmet needs

- The inner critic: Tries to protect you from failure and rejection but often becomes harsh and limiting

- The perfectionist: Drives you toward excellence but can create paralysis and never-enough thinking

- The rebel: Fights against control and conformity but can sabotage your goals

- The caretaker: Wants to help and please others but may neglect your needs

- The wise elder: Holds your deepest wisdom and perspective but may be drowned out by louder voices

When you're unconscious of these parts, they often work against each other. The perfectionist might set impossible standards while the rebel sabotages any attempt to meet them.

The Round Table visualization:

Imagine sitting at a round table, or around a fire, with different versions of yourself – perhaps an inner child, wise elder, rebellious teen, or inner critic.

Get to know these characters with curiosity and compassion. Listen to their advice, complaints, desires, and aversions. The more you connect with your internal parts, the more whole, connected, and embodied you'll feel and live.

My story:

I've worked extensively with my inner teen. This part of me gets ice-cold angry when I ignore my heart's truth. As I acknowledge her pain and needs, the less she hijacks my nervous system. She's become an important signal that I'm out of alignment. The sooner I listen to her cues, the more I stay embodied and present.

The goal isn't to eliminate any parts but to create awareness and connection with them. Like a good conductor with an orchestra, learn to give each part its moment to be heard while maintaining overall direction and flow. This creates a sense of wholeness and harmony that's otherwise impossible.

The practice:

Close your eyes and imagine your inner round table. Who shows up? What are their names? What do they want you to know? Create ongoing dialogue with these parts of yourself. They're not problems to fix but aspects to integrate. You might be surprised by who shows up at your table. You might find parts of yourself that you have long forgotten or disowned. You might find parts of yourself that are angry, sad, or scared. And you might find parts of yourself that are wise, loving, and powerful. All of these parts belong. All of these parts have an impact. And all of these parts have a key to your functional embodiment.

Living your embodied life

These five pathways work together to create functional embodiment – a way of living that honors your body's wisdom, embraces your emotions, harnesses the power of your thinking, integrates your inner characters, and supports conscious choices for your well-being. Rather than following external rules, you learn to trust your internal guidance system and respond with care.

This creates a ripple effect: when you operate from embodied presence, you naturally want to nourish yourself with choices that support vitality. You crave movement that energizes you, relationships that feed you, and spend your time in ways that align with your values.

You become your own body expert – someone who trusts their internal signals and makes aligned choices. You are the creator of your own experience. The guidance you seek isn't outside of you – it's within you, waiting to be acknowledged and honored.

Functional embodiment is not a one-time fix. It is a lifelong practice. There will be times when you feel disconnected, and there will be times when you feel deeply embodied. The goal is not to be perfect, but to be present. The goal is not to eliminate your struggles, but to learn how to navigate them with grace, instinct, and wisdom. The goal is to come home to your body wisdom, again and again and again.

May you feel empowered, enlivened, connected, calm, and trusting.

Final thoughts

Be patient with yourself as you develop these new patterns. Recognize and celebrate each moment of listening to your body knowing, like I did when my baby was nestled in my arms, because celebrating builds momentum. Trust that you have signals and cues within you to create a life of clarity, calm, and connection

You're already home. You've always been home. These embodiment tools simply help you remember what your body has never forgotten. Welcome home to your own wisdom. Welcome home to your body. Welcome home to yourself.

Key takeaways to implement

As you consider implementing these practices, trust your inner guidance about where to begin. Your body will tell you which pathway calls to you first. Honor that instinct.

* Honor your body signals, cues, and instincts:

  * When your body says no to water, food, or medication – honor the cue. Your body's wisdom is refined by millions of years of evolution.

  * Get to know the thoughts, beliefs, and expectations in your supercomputer mind. Write them down and look at them objectively. Notice their cascade effect on your emotions and behavior.

    * Remember: you have the option to choose your thoughts and make clear requests.

* The snacking/scrolling challenge:

  * For one day, flag every time you reach for food or your phone. Ask: "Am I doing this to avoid an emotion?" If so, make the choice to lean in and feel that emotion instead. Allow it space in your metaphorical car.

* Implement mindful check-ins:

  * When wanting to shift habits, regularly ask: "How do I want to feel in two hours? Tomorrow morning? Ten years from now?" Make decisions considering how you want to feel long term.

* Find your growth community:

  * Consider joining a local integration group or finding growth-focused humans to be around. Growth is contagious and encouraging, especially when integrating 'the work' feels challenging.

Thank you for allowing me to share this journey with you.

About the author

Chandra Zas has dedicated her life to helping people reconnect with their internal wisdom for sustainable well-being. With nearly three decades of experience in somatic practices and consciousness work, Chandra bridges ancient wisdom traditions with modern psychological understanding to create practical pathways for transformation.

Currently serving as an integration circle facilitator with Sierra Psychedelic Society, in Reno, Nevada, Chandra supports community members in integrating profound experiences into daily life.

Her training includes certifications as a yoga teacher, massage therapist, and Ayurveda practitioner, complemented by years of immersive study at institutions including Esalen Institute, BodyMind Restoration Retreats, and Quiet Star. This diverse background allows her to offer a uniquely integrated approach to healing that honors both the body's intelligence and the mind's capacity for conscious choice.

Learn more about Chandra's work, offerings, and philosophy at chandrazas.com. You can also find her on most social media @ChandraZas. She welcomes your connection.

chandrazas.com

@ChandraZas

Part Two

Functional Body Care

Nikia works with professional athletes — my favorite source for cutting-edge health approaches. I was thrilled when she agreed to write about the minimal effective dose for fitness, shifting the paradigm from "push harder" to "train smarter" for sustainable physical wellbeing.

Her grounded perspective on how exercise affects hormonal balance has transformed my understanding of workout energy management.

— Book momma Chandra

1

Minimum Effective Dose: A Return to Holistic Movement

Dr. Nikia Evans

There comes a moment, often quiet, sometimes painful, when we realize the way we've been moving is no longer working. First, the body whispers. Then it aches. Then it demands. Not for more reps, more goals, more plans — but for something more ancient: rhythm, restoration, and reverence.

Paracelsus once wrote, "The dose makes the poison." But in movement, as in medicine, that same law governs healing. Too little, and we lose vitality. Too much, and we tip into depletion. The power lies not in doing more, but in finding the rhythm that restores.

This insight forms the foundation of what I call the Minimum Effective Dose (MED) framework. It is a way to reclaim movement as medicine. When we move too much, too often, or without rhythm, we risk draining our reserves. But when we do too little, we stagnate, losing resilience and biological intelligence. The MED framework is not a training plan or a challenge. It's a recalibration, a remembering.

Rooted in circadian science, ancestral patterns, and fascial physiology — and shaped by years spent moving through recovery, elite sport, clinical spaces, and deep nature — this framework invites you to ask: *What's just enough?* What's the least you can do to stay deeply well, and, paradoxically, regenerate more fully? This is not about intensity. It's about integrity. Done with care, the Minimum Effective Dose (MED) becomes

27

the most potent medicine — not because it's extreme, but because it's sustainable. It's something your body remembers — how to come home, how to heal, how to begin again. The encoded rhythm of repair will lead you home, if only you let it.

This approach was born not in a lab, but in the quiet reckoning of my own healing — when years of pushing harder stopped working. When I had to re-learn how to flourish within the rhythm of my own body — in relationship with nature, not in defiance of it. Today, I am a physician, an athlete, a researcher, and a guide — but more than that, I am someone who had to unlearn performance as identity and relearn presence as medicine. It took shape through seasons of guiding hundreds of elite athletes, walking beside people in their healing, recovering from injury and illness myself, and continually honoring what it means to come back home — to my own body, again and again.

If you choose to keep reading, I'll walk you through the rhythms that changed everything — and perhaps, they'll help you return to something you've been missing too.

Minimum: The wisdom of enough

The first principle of healing is simplicity. In a culture that equates health with hustle, we often overlook the quiet, potent wisdom of restraint. Yet some of the most transformative shifts happen not through doing more, but through doing just enough, again and again, with reverence.

To honor the minimum is not to settle. It is to subtract the unnecessary until what remains is deeply life-giving. A breath. A step. A return to what your body recognizes as home: sunlight, gravity, warmth, breath, stillness, sensation. These are not luxuries. They are the foundations of regeneration — the biological rhythms that shaped us, and the ones we need to truly return to health.

In the MED framework, minimums are not arbitrary checklists, they are signals. Signals to your nervous system that you are safe. To your hormones that you are steady. To your tissues that you are ready to repair, not react. These rhythms give your body the message that life is not something to muscle through, but something to move through — fluidly, wisely, without bracing.

And here's the paradox: when you honor the minimums, your capacity grows, your energy returns, inflammation quiets. The body starts to trust itself again.

This is not a hack. It's an invitation to come home to coherence.

Ask yourself: What rhythms make you feel human again? What is just enough to soften your edges, to steady your breath, to remind your body that it belongs?

This is where the five rituals begin: **walk, restore, play, train, and recover**. They are not rules, but remembrances. Not another performance to perfect, but a way of living that regenerates what was never lost, only silenced.

If you do nothing but the three minimums — mostly outside, mostly in sunlight, mostly in rhythm — your body will begin to transform.

1. Walk: Return to the Earth

Before training plans and performance metrics, before shoes or streets or gyms, we walked.

We walked for water, for food, for each other. We walked to grieve. To heal. To feel the wind. Walking is our first medicine. It shaped our brains, aligned our spines, sculpted our breath. Bipedal movement is what shifted us upright, attuned us to the world and made us human.

And it's still what brings us back.

When your body feels fragmented or fatigued, when your nervous system is on edge, when your thoughts feel tangled — walk. It is the simplest, most powerful way to restore coherence. Your lymph begins to flow. Your spine begins to self-correct. Cortisol drops, blood sugar stabilizes, sex hormones recalibrate, mitochondria wake up. You don't have to optimize this. Your body already knows what to do because it's encoded in your gait.

This is why walking is not a warm-up — it is our first medicine. It's the pulse your body remembers when all else has failed. Within the MED framework, walking forms the foundation of recovery, rhythm, and return. It regulates without force. It restores without depletion. It is, quite literally, how we come home.

So walk for around 12,000 steps a day, five days per week, which is roughly 90 to 120 minutes depending on your stride. Whenever possible walk barefoot or in minimalist shoes on uneven ground. But don't walk for numbers. Walk for rhythm. Walk for breath. Walk for clarity. If you only do this — consistently, in nature, and under real light — your body will begin to regenerate.

Walking regulates the vagus nerve, hydrates the fascia, stabilizes joints, and supports circadian and hormonal balance. It is gentle enough to do every day, powerful enough to transform your physiology, and simple enough to keep you from getting lost in the noise of modern movement culture.

This is not about productivity. It's about presence. To walk with awareness is to remember that your body was never broken — just rushed. Just disconnected.

To be human is to walk. To meet the earth with every step. To carry memory in your fascia, intelligence in your rhythm, and reverence in your stride.

2. Restore: Unwind the tensions

If walking restores rhythm, *restore* reclaims suppleness — the fluid intelligence beneath strength. It is not a stretch. Not a cooldown. Not an afterthought. It is the sacred space where your body unravels what it has been holding too tightly, for too long.

These are not workouts. They are un-layerings.

Every clenched jaw, every tight hip, every held breath is a message — not just of physical tension, but of accumulated emotion, bracing, and unsafety. Rituals of restoration meet these signals with presence, not pressure. Here, we soften instead of stretch. We listen instead of fix. We make space, not demands.

I guide clients to explore three primary modalities:

- **Fascial flow** — Spiraling, intuitive sequences drawn from yoga, tai-chi, Pilates, primal patterns, and somatic traditions. These aren't about flexibility; they're about fluidity. Rehydrating tissue. Restoring feel. Re-patterning motion from the inside out. This is how fascia becomes expressive again — not through force, but through rhythm and hydration.

- **Manual myofascial care** — Using your hands, tools, or breath as instruments of dialogue. Think gua sha, scraping, gentle compression, manual therapy, or ball work, not as aggression on tissues, but as communication. Over time, you'll learn the language of your adhesions and how to meet them with curiosity.

- **Targeted breathwork** — Breath directed to tension sites, layered with gentle movement or touch. A tight hip often speaks to diaphragm collapse, pelvic floor bracing, or old survival signals. Breathing here, with softness, is not just physiological, it's deeply somatic.

These practices are not passive. They're participatory. You're not fixing your body, you're partnering with it. Listening. Softening. Repatterning. Each session teaches your nervous system that sensation is not a threat, but information. That movement can be safe again. That your body is trustworthy.

Start with 10–25 minutes, two or three times per week. Don't aim for heroic efforts, instead aim for repetition, rhythm, and respect. The nervous system doesn't respond to once-a-month breakthroughs. It responds to rituals of safety. The kind that says, "*You're not under attack. You can soften now. You can let go.*"

Restore practices are particularly powerful for recalibrating hormones and healing chronic depletion. When you shift out of survival mode, cortisol normalizes, insulin sensitivity improves, progesterone and estrogen return to equilibrium. Recovery accelerates. Sleep deepens. Inflammation cools.

I've seen athletes recover from long-standing injury, not by isolating a single muscle, but by restoring coherence through myofascial care. I've seen new mothers reconnect to their core without crunches. I've seen people cry, laugh, and finally exhale — not because a stretch was deep, but because their body was finally seen.

Restore is a ceremony of return. A ritual of softness. A pulse of self-trust. It is how we remind the body that healing is not earned through effort, but allowed through deeper listening.

3. Play: Reclaim the wild

Where *walk* reconnects us with rhythm and *restore* invites us to release, *play* reminds us of who we are beneath performance — unpredictable, adaptive, and wild.

Play is not a luxury, it is a lost language. One that speaks directly to your nervous system, your fascia, and your spirit. It rewires your relationship to movement, not through metrics or mastery, but through curiosity. Through joy. Through a kind of sacred chaos.

Play is where your body remembers it is a creature of the wild — built for spontaneity, creativity, and connection. I've spent decades in structured training environments, and I've learned that without *play*, performance becomes pathology. *Play* isn't childish, it's primal. It teaches reaction, risk, and resilience. It reprograms stress through joy and awakens agility without forcing it.

This isn't just fun, it's functional neurobiology. *Play* stimulates the cerebellum, improving balance and coordination. It lights up the prefrontal cortex, enhancing problem-solving, emotional regulation, and creativity. It interrupts chronic threat detection and reintroduces lightness into the fascia. It teaches the brain to process unpredictability — a skill more vital than ever in a world of constant change.

It also transforms stress. Where cortisol once spiked, oxytocin and dopamine flow. The body softens. The mind sharpens. You stop performing — and start participating. Fully, instinctively, without outcome.

There are no rules, only invitations. Try skipping down a trail. Dance in your kitchen. Toss a ball and chase it like a child. Balance on rocks or fallen logs. Join a spontaneous game. Wrestle gently with a loved one. Do cartwheels. Make up a movement game with your kids. Let yourself be moved by joy rather than agenda.

In my years coaching athletes, working with patients, and finding my own way back from burnout, I've seen this again and again: *play* reanimates curiosity and restores the body's trust in movement. Not because it's productive, but because it's primal. It awakens a part of you that's been waiting — beneath the metrics and mandates — the part not here to win, but to feel, to explore, and to belong.

To play is to remember what it means to move, not for the sake of progress, but for the sheer aliveness of it.

Effective: Align with the body's intelligence

To be *effective* is not to be efficient. It is to be attuned. It means listening to the body's signals and moving in ways that support strength, adaptability, and growth.

We are not machines to optimize. We are ecosystems that are living, cyclical, and intelligent. True effectiveness emerges when movement matches biology. When rhythm and rest, challenge and recovery, and are in right relationship.

The most effective movement isn't the most extreme — it's the most coherent. It builds capacity without collapse. It strengthens not just muscle, but metabolism, focus, and flow. And perhaps most importantly, it reveals what the body can do — not just what it can survive.

The five rituals — *walk, restore, play, train, recover* — are effective because they're biologically familiar. They're embedded in our nervous systems, fascia, and hormonal rhythms. They support integration across systems — from skeletal alignment to mitochondrial function.

Effectiveness also means precision: knowing what to do, when to do it, and when to stop. It's not about maximizing effort but about meeting your body with clarity and care. That's what creates real change, and the kind that lasts.

This is where the *train* ritual begins. Importantly, not from exhaustion, but from readiness. When the first three rituals have grounded you in rhythm and responsiveness, you are ready to expand. Ready to train not to prove yourself, but to express who you truly are.

4. Train: Reawaken the primal codes

Training is not required for health. But when done with rhythm, it becomes a catalyst — a way to refine systems, enhance expression, and rise to challenge with grace. It builds upon the foundations laid by walking, restoring, and playing, not as a separate pursuit but a natural expansion. When the body is regulated, nourished, and curious, it is ready to grow.

The most resilient systems are the most adaptive. Effective *training* engages a spectrum: unilateral strength, split stance work, rotational dynamics, and integrated locomotion. This isn't about building a bigger engine, it's about becoming a more intelligent mover. Intelligent *training* also avoids the common trap of repetition without range. Overuse of narrow joint angles — the same bilateral lifts or linear cardio — leads to dysfunction, not durability. Instead, training should reflect our full biological blueprint: crawling, climbing, throwing, running, and striking. These patterns don't just build muscle, they reawaken coordination, elasticity, and neuroendocrine integrity. Train not as a grind, but as a refinement. Of breath under tension. Of force through fascia. Of integrity across systems from neuromuscular firing to metabolic flexibility. Your training should not reduce you to tightness and fatigue. It should reveal your coherence.

Choose two to three of these primal patterns each session — crawling, climbing, throwing, running, striking — and spend 30 to 50 minutes working within them. Explore not for reps, but for reconnection. Crawl to reawaken coordination. Slam or throw to build power. Swing from bars to restore grip, gaze, and gait. Relearn them the way a child does: through curiosity, adaptability, and full-body feedback. Let terrain, tempo, and tension be your teachers.

If your goals are more specific, such as returning from injury, building sport specific power, increasing speed, or preventing burnout, consider seeking guidance. A skilled practitioner can align your training with your physiology, prevent overload, and tailor intensity to your rhythm. One of the most powerful acts of self-stewardship is knowing when to ask for support.

Train not to fix what's broken, but to explore what's possible. Let your movement become an expression of readiness — of rhythm restored, of strength reclaimed, of a system no longer in defense, but in flow.

Dose: The art of listening

Dose is not just about how much. It's about when, why, and in response to what. It is the rhythm beneath the rhythm, the signal that tells your body how to adapt.

In pharmacology, the right medicine at the wrong dose becomes a toxin. The same is true in movement. Even the most sacred rituals I've outlined so far, such as walking, restoring, playing, and training, can become depleting when mismatched to your capacity.

That's what makes *dose* the intelligence within the MED framework. It's the part that listens. That adjusts. That gives these same five rituals a different tone depending on the season you're in. It's what makes them feel like medicine in one phase of life, and maintenance in another. This is where the shift happens, from "What should I do?" to "What do I need, right now?" To dose movement wisely, you must become a student of your own patterns — of your cycle, your symptoms, your sleep, your stress, and your season. This is not self-optimization. It's self-stewardship. A living relationship with effort and ease.

Done well, *dose* doesn't just help you do more. It helps you sense more — and choose more skillfully. It's how the same input becomes gentler when you're depleted, sharper when you're ready, and more effective in the long run. Dose is how we honor the complexity of being human — not by pushing through, but by tuning in.

5. Recover: Honor the cycle

Recovery is not the opposite of training, it is the completion of it. This is where effort transmutes into growth, where strength integrates, and where the body absorbs what it has been given. It is in these moments of stillness that hormones recalibrate, tissues repair, and the psyche begins to quiet again. Some of the most elite performers, and the most grounded healers I've known, share a single truth: you cannot keep outputting and expect coherence. *Recovery* is not optional, it is essential.

Yet this is often the ritual we resist most. In a culture that equates rest with weakness, we override the very signals designed to protect us. But true *recovery* is not passive. It is alive with recalibration. It is where the nervous system reorients, where the immune system fortifies, and where the subtle systems of fascia, hormones, and mitochondria can come back into rhythm. It is not doing nothing. It is doing the most important thing: allowing integration.

To *recover* well is to say no — not from avoidance, but from wisdom. To wait — not from fear, but from trust. It is where you sit in the stillness and let the earth catch up to your cells. Where you lay down your striving and remember that regeneration is not something to earn but something you allow. Honor your sleep, your cycle, your sunlight, your silence. Let your rhythms lead. Step back from the metrics and the noise and watch what happens when your body is given the time it actually needs. *Recovery* is not about bouncing back — it's about coming back deeper, clearer, and more whole.

This is movement, not as punishment, but as prayer. Not as performance, but as presence. *Recovery* is the final pulse in the rhythm — the exhale that makes all the effort worthwhile. It is here, in this quiet, that you return to yourself.

Welcome home.

Key takeaways to implement

* *Walk* daily (aim for ~12,000 steps, 5x/week), ideally in nature and sunlight.

* *Restore* tension and nervous system tone 2 to 3x/week through fascia-focused movement, breath, and soft-tissue care.

* *Play* regularly — invite spontaneity, joy, and curiosity back into movement.

Remember, if you do nothing but the minimums — walking, restoring, and playing — mostly outdoors, under real sunlight, your body will re-generate more than most training plans can offer. Training is not required for healing. It's for expansion. If you're still rebuilding, stay with the earlier rituals. Let rhythm and nature be your medicine. The body knows what to do with them.

About the author

Dr. Nikia Evans, MD, MS-AKP, is a physician, researcher, and human performance coach passionate about reimagining movement as medicine—not just for performance, but as a path to resilience. Her work integrates fascia-informed movement, hormone support, energy system development, metabolic priming, and nervous system regulation to help athletes and active humans reconnect with their inherent capacity to heal, adapt, and thrive. Connect with her on socials @itsthatgoodmedicine or at www.itsthatgoodmedicine.com for resources and deeper guidance on movement, recovery, and coming home to your body's innate wisdom.

itsthatgoodmedicine.com

@itsthatgoodmedicine

I was told that I had to meet Keaton. He was giving a keynote on breath and sleep at a local startup conference. Sleep was one of the topics I specifically sought for this book. His expertise in breathwork and sleep optimization offers practical solutions to foundational health challenges that many of us face in our busy modern lives.

You can skip on food and feel ok, but missing sleep wreaks havoc.

— *Book momma Chandra*

2

Breath and Sleep: The Missing Links to Your Foundation

Keaton Lynn

As I watched my nephew's belly rise, I noticed how perfect his breath was. He was eight months old at the time, lying beside his twin sister in their mother's arms. Both fast asleep, their bellies rose and fell in unison. Their mouths were closed, their inhales and exhales silent. Their chests rose only slightly. Their shoulders stayed still.

The first thing we do in this world is breathe. It's the sign of life doctors and nurses look for — and the first thing a mother wants to hear. Breath is the foundation of our being. You can go roughly three weeks without food, three days without water, but only about three minutes without air. And yet, for many of us, breath has become a background process. We forget that it's the only system in the body that is both autonomic, like our heartbeat, and somatic, like moving your finger.

Today, most people lose proper breathing techniques somewhere along the way. We go from breathing perfectly, like my niece and nephew, to dysfunctional patterns. I see this all the time in my work with athletes and first responders. Helping them reconnect with their breath improves performance.

In *What Doesn't Kill Us*, investigative journalist Scott Carney tries to disprove the work of Wim Hof. What makes the book powerful is that Scott enters the story a skeptic. He wants to expose Wim as a fraud. But through his journey, he experiences something profound. He ends up climbing Mt. Kilimanjaro in just shorts and no shirt — in a single day.

That book made me think. I remember putting it down, sitting cross-legged on the floor, and asking myself: *Is my stomach supposed to expand or shrink when I inhale?* How could I not know the answer to that? This is my body, and I breathe over 16,000 times a day — and I wasn't even sure if my stomach should go out or in on an inhale.

I was in great shape. Training twice a day. Working long hours. I was competing in one of the most demanding environments of my life. I had played collegiate water polo and swam competitively. In high school, I was an All-American who played ten seasons of sports. And yet, I had never really learned how to breathe.

That moment shifted everything. It started my journey into breathwork.

Activity: How is your breath?

Take a moment. Stand in front of a mirror. Inhale deeply and just watch your body. What moves? Your chest? Your belly? Your shoulders? Do you breathe in through your nose or mouth? Do you feel better, worse, or no change at all?

This is real-time feedback. Your breath is a mirror for performance, recovery, mindset, even how your face will age. It affects your smile, your stress, and your health span.

What is breath?

Pranayama is the Sanskrit word for breath and has been practiced for centuries. From ancient warriors preparing for battle to monks in deep meditation, breath has always been a tool for control and clarity.

Breath is the only system in the body governed by both the autonomic nervous system (which controls things like digestion and heart rate) and the somatic nervous system (which governs voluntary movement). That means it can run automatically, but you can also take control of it at any moment.

You can shift your breathing pattern with awareness, and let it go again. Breath is a two-way communication system between the body and the brain. Jesse Coomer, in his book *The Language of Breath*, describes breath as a language — one that can be listened to, learned, and eventually spoken.

Breathing is the gas exchange between your external world and your internal one. You breathe in oxygen and exhale carbon dioxide. Humans are carbon-based lifeforms, but oxygen is our engine. It's our Origin 1 healer. Without oxygen, we can't repair, recover, or perform. Down to the cellular level — the Krebs cycle — oxygen is essential.

Question to reflect on:
If I'm constantly breathing wrong,
will that affect my body's energy output?

Absolutely. Your breath pattern affects your heart rate. Inhale, and your heart rate rises. Exhale, and it falls. If you're over-breathing all day, your heart rate is staying elevated. That affects blood pressure, hormones, mental clarity, stress response — everything. It's all connected.

Biomechanics

From birth to about age five, children learn by moving. Then, they start school. They go from crawling and playing to sitting in chairs for hours a day. The natural mechanics of breath shift. Shoulders start rising. Breathing becomes shallow. Mouth breathing takes over.

Understanding how you lost your breath is step one. From there, you can start to retrain it. And when you do, everything improves: performance, energy, clarity, mood.

Mirror check-in

Remember the mirror activity? Picture yourself doing that thousands of times a day. Your breath is your foundation. What did your shoulders do? Your belly? Did they move?

Breathing well while calm builds the mechanics you'll rely on under stress. It creates a baseline.

The BOLT Score

Let's measure. This is your **BOLT Score** (Blood Oxygen Level Test). It's not a max breath hold. Here's how to take it:

1. Sit down, relax. Grab your phone stopwatch.

2. Take a normal inhale. Then a soft exhale. Now hold your breath.

3. Start the timer as you hold.

4. Stop the timer the moment you feel the *urge* to breathe.

How to score it:

- Less than 10 seconds: Poor breathing, needs work.

- 10—20 seconds: Room for improvement.

- 20—30 seconds: Solid. Good biomechanics.

- 30—40+ seconds: Great oxygen efficiency.

Optimal breath

Ideal breathing starts at the diaphragm — a muscle below your lungs. When you inhale, it contracts downward, creating pressure that draws air into your lungs.

Pressure is the key. At sea level, it's easier to breathe. At altitude, it's harder because the atmospheric pressure is lower — not because there's less oxygen.

Gas exchange happens in the **bottom third** of your lungs, where the highest density of alveoli live. If you're not breathing deep, you're losing access to most of your oxygen capacity.

Your rib cage should expand. Your intercostal muscles should activate. Your lower back should press into the floor. Finally, your chest rises slightly — not your shoulders. That's optimal breathing.

Ocean breathing visualization

Think of breath like a wave:

- It builds from your belly.

- Grows up into your ribs.

- Peaks in the chest.

- Crashes in the exhale.

Breathe like a wave. Feel it rise and fall. This visualization helps your body learn the language of breath.

Where is your breath now?

Let's find your starting point. Lay on your back and slowly breathe in. Feel your lower torso expand — in the front, sides, and lower back. Then into your ribs. Finally, into your chest. As you exhale, your chest falls, your ribs soften, and your belly sinks.

How do you feel now? Calm? Relaxed? Lighter?

You probably feel better because of two key nerves: the vagus nerve and the phrenic nerve. The vagus controls your emotional state and parasympathetic response. The slower you breathe, the more relaxed you become. The phrenic nerve tells your diaphragm when to contract and release. These nerves, and how you breathe, shape your state.

The problem with over-breathing

Modern life puts our nervous system on high alert. Fast breathing. Shallow breaths. Always "on." This chronic stress loop hijacks our breath and keeps us in a sympathetic state — fight or flight — even when we're just sitting at a desk.

Athletes, high performers, and busy professionals often skip the fundamentals. They train hard. Push harder. But without mastering the breath, they're missing a massive piece of the puzzle.

Breathing is the gateway to managing stress, regulating emotion, and unlocking peak performance. Yet most people are stuck over-breathing — taking short, rapid breaths through the mouth.

The average American breathes about 16.7 times per minute. But optimal function happens at 6 to 8 breaths per minute. That's a huge difference. Imagine your engine revving in the red all day. It burns out. Over time, that leads to chronic stress, fatigue, and disease.

Think about it like your dream car — let's say a Mustang GT500. Would you drive it at max RPM all day, every day? No chance. But that's exactly what many people do with their breath. They stay revved up without even realizing it.

Learning to downshift matters. You need to know when to push and when to pull back. When to breathe hard, and when to breathe slow. Your breath can help you flip the switch.

Activity: Inner awareness check-in

Lie down. Close your eyes. Breathe naturally. Now, scan your body:

- What do you feel in your back? Your hips? Your chest?

- Where is your mind?

- Are you thinking clearly or drifting?

- Can you feel your heartbeat in your fingertips?

Now shift into active breath control:

- Inhale through your nose for 6 seconds.

- Exhale through your nose for 6 seconds.

This even cadence activates your parasympathetic nervous system. It keeps you calm, yet alert. It's perfect for waking up gently or easing into your day with intention.

Notice how your body responds. Do you fee more grounded? Are your thoughts clearer? This is the language of your breath taking shape.

Now ask yourself:

- Are you breathing into your belly?
- Are your ribs expanding?
- Can you feel your lower back pressing into the ground?
- Is your chest rising last, like a wave cresting?

This is optimal. This is your new baseline.

Breath and sleep: The missing link

Now that you understand the power of breath, let's talk about its secret partner: sleep.

Breathing and sleep go hand in hand. You can survive poor food for weeks. Poor hydration for days. But just one night of poor sleep and you feel it everywhere.

Sleep is the most overlooked recovery tool.
And breath is your access point to better sleep.

Think about it. Even in the days of saber-toothed tigers and cave danger, humans risked everything to sleep. That's how vital it is. Yet today, most adults average less than 6.5 hours per night and wonder why they feel drained.

Before we get into the tactics, ask yourself:

- Do you feel rested?
- Do you dread going to bed?
- Are you wired at night but tired in the morning?

Let's change that — starting tonight.

Circadian Rhythm: Your 24-hour clock

Your body runs on rhythm. Here's a rough timeline of how it flows:

9 p.m. - Melatonin begins to rise.

10 p.m. - Ideal bedtime.

11 p.m. - Deep sleep begins.

2 a.m. - REM sleep phase.

4 a.m. - Body temperature hits its lowest point.

6 a.m. - Blood pressure rises.

7 a.m. - Cortisol spikes to wake you.

9 a.m. - Brain is primed for deep work.

3:30 p.m. - Peak reaction time.

5:30 p.m. - Strength output peaks.

7 p.m. - Body temperature hits daily high.

When you align your life to this rhythm, everything gets easier: energy, focus, workouts, even digestion.

The five sleep fundamentals

1. **Light:** Dim your lights after sunset. Use red light or candlelight if possible. In the morning, get outside within 30 minutes of waking. Light is your most powerful circadian tool.

2. **Noise:** Keep your room under 35db if possible. If ambient noise is unavoidable, use earplugs or a white noise machine to avoid sudden disturbances.

3. **Temperature:** Keep your room cool: 62—69°F is ideal. You can always add a blanket, but your face should stay cool for optimal breathing and thermoregulation.

4. **Bed Use:** Your bed is for sleep and sex. That's it. No phones. No tv. No late-night scrolling. Your brain needs to associate your bed with deep rest.

5. **Breath:** Nasal breathing at night is critical. Mouth breathing leads to snoring, poor oxygen absorption, and disrupted recovery. Your breath is the silent healer during sleep.

Want a shortcut? Check out my "Trybe Sleep Kit" on Amazon. It includes all the essentials for light, breath, and comfort.

When life happens: Sleep on shift

Let's be real — life doesn't always follow the perfect schedule. You might be a firefighter, a nurse, a parent, or someone grinding through late-night workouts just to stay afloat. That's okay. This approach isn't about guilt — it's about tools.

So, let's say you finish your only available workout at 9 p.m. You go hard: warm-up, heavy lift, a full *MetCon, and sprints. You're buzzing with adrenaline, and your heart rate is sky-high. But you also want deep sleep to recover. (*MetCon stands for Metabolic Conditioning. It is a type of workout that will exert your cardiovascular system (getting you out of breath) and will also get your heart rate up, increasing your overall level of fitness.)

Here's the blueprint to shift gears from performance to rest:

Step 1: Gear down

Right after your workout, cool down with gentle cardio (bike, jog, or row) and begin downshifting your breath:

- From Gear 4 (heavy mouth breathing)

- To Gear 3 (inhale nose, exhale mouth)

- Then to Gear 2 (inhale nose, exhale nose)

- Finally Gear 1 (slow nasal only, calm state)

Step 2: Floor work + Breathing protocols

Find a quiet spot. Lie down. Close your eyes. Start with 3 minutes of double nasal inhales, followed by long, slow exhales through your mouth. Then shift into a 4:0:8:0 breath pattern (inhale 4, exhale 8, no holds). Do this for another 3 minutes.

Step 3: Post-workout recovery nutrition

If you didn't eat before, prep a light meal high in carbs with moderate protein (about 30g). If you did eat, a small shake or light snack is enough. Avoid heavy meals close to bedtime.

Step 4: Shift the environment

- Keep lights low or off
- Avoid screens
- Take a warm shower

Step 5: Night routine wind-down

Start your bedtime routine in dim lighting. Journal, prep for the next day, or read away from your bed. When your body feels heavy and ready, get into bed and allow yourself to fall asleep.

Now contrast that with what most people do:

- Bright lights
- Doom scrolling
- Heavy meals
- No breath regulation
- High cortisol before bed

The result? Poor sleep. Elevated stress. Frustrated mornings. You don't reset.

Your breath is your tool to downshift. To recover. To reset the system for tomorrow.

The Gear System: Breathe in Gears

Just like your car has gears, so does your body. Use them wisely.

Gear 1: Everyday life. Calm. Walking. Working. Breathing in and out through the nose. This is your baseline. You should spend 80 percent of your day here.

Gear 2: Zone 2 cardio. Slight exertion but sustainable. Inhale and exhale through the nose. Some strain is okay. You should spend 10 percent of your day here.

Gear 3: High intensity. You're working hard. Inhale through the nose, exhale through the mouth. Think: HIIT or MetCon-style training. This is about 5 percent of your day.

Gear 4: Max output. Sprinting. Peak performance. Inhale and exhale through the mouth. You just need oxygen. Spend the least amount of time here — about 5 percent max.

Use your gears intentionally:

- Warm up in Gear 2

- Shift to Gear 3 before go-time

- Go full send in Gear 4

- Downshift: Gear 3 → Gear 2 → Gear 1

Mastering your breath in each gear gives you control over your body, mind, and performance.

Breathing protocol library

This appendix is your breathwork toolkit — simple patterns you can use to shift your state anytime, anywhere. Each one is listed as a ratio: **Inhale: Hold (inhaled): Exhale: Hold (exhaled)**. Customize the timing based on your level.

Box Breathing (4:4:4:4)

For calm focus. Great for starting the day, resetting under stress, or entering a mindful state. Beginners can use 3-second counts; advanced users can push to 6 or 7.

Apnea Breathing (4:8:4:0 or 4:0:4:8)

Used for athletic warm-ups. The first version emphasizes inhale holds; the second emphasizes exhale holds. Try both and see which works better for your prep.

Bedtime Breath (4:0:8:0)

Your go-to for winding down. Long exhale, no holds. This one resets the system and calms the nervous system. For even deeper rest, try 3:7:8:0.

Power Breathing (2:0:1:0)

Need a boost? Use this short, sharp breath cycle to ramp up energy.

Ocean Breathing (8:0:8:0)

Inhale slowly through your nose, exhale slowly as if fogging a mirror. A great protocol for morning grounding or nighttime wind-down.

Low-High Breath (Body Awareness Practice)

Lie down with one hand on your belly, one on your chest. Breathe first into your lower torso. Feel your stomach rise, ribs expand, and lower back press into the floor. Then try a chest-only breath to compare. End by combining both for a full-body wave.

Triangle Breathing (3:3:3:0)

Great for foundational practice. You can move the "hold" to any point. Inhale-hold-exhale, or inhale-exhale-hold. Simple and powerful.

Cadence Breathing (3:3:6:3 or 1:1:2:1)

A structured, parasympathetic-focused breath. Good for recovery or post-workout.

Fire Breathing (1:0:1:0)

Fast and powerful. Use with caution for short bursts only. It's meant to wake you up fast or shift gears rapidly.

Final thoughts: Inspiration to breathe

So, what more can I say to get you to breathe intentionally?

What if I told you your facial structure can change? Your emotional control can sharpen? Your immune response can strengthen?

What if you could prevent disease, improve focus, and feel more present, all from something you already do 16,000 times a day?

This approach isn't just about knowledge. It's about awareness. About reclaiming a forgotten language your body has always spoken. Breathing well isn't a trick. It's a foundation. And now you have the tools to build it.

Your breath impacts your performance, your recovery, your aging, your focus, your sleep, and your emotional health. And it's available to you, right now, for free.

So, take a breath.

Now take another.

You're already on your way.

Key takeaways to implement

❋ Implement the Gear System for breath control throughout your day.

Identify which "gear" you're in throughout the day:

◇ Gear 1 (80 percent of day): Nasal breathing in/out during rest, work, and daily activities.

◇ Gear 2 (10 percent of day): Nasal breathing in/out during light exercise (walking, easy cardio).

◇ Gear 3 (5 percent of day): Nasal in, mouth out during moderate-intensity activities.

◇ Gear 4 (5 percent of day): Mouth breathing in/out only during maximum exertion.

❋ Practice intentional "downshifting" after exercise or stress:

◇ From Gear 4 → 3 → 2 → 1 using progressively slower breathing

◇ Use the 4:0:8:0 pattern (inhale 4 seconds, exhale 8 seconds) to downshift quickly

❋ Set a reminder on your phone to check your breathing pattern every 2 hours.

Implementation Trigger: Create a small card with the four gears listed to keep in your wallet or on your desk as a reference.

❋ Establish a breath-based sleep preparation routine

◇ Begin your sleep preparation 30 minutes before bedtime.

◇ Dim lights and avoid screens to support natural melatonin production.

◇ Perform 3 minutes of the "Bedtime Breath" protocol (4:0:8:0 pattern).

▪ Inhale through nose for 4 seconds.

- Exhale through nose for 8 seconds (twice as long as inhale).

- No breath holds.

- Ensure your bedroom is cool (62-69°F) and quiet.

- Focus on nasal breathing as you fall asleep (use mouth tape if needed).

- Upon waking, get natural sunlight within 30 minutes to reset your circadian rhythm.

Implementation Trigger: Set an alarm 30 minutes before your ideal bedtime labeled "Begin Sleep Breath Protocol."

About the author

Keaton Lynn is a veteran, adventurer, and lifelong learner with over a decade in lifestyle performance. With multiple certifications and an obsession with breathwork and biomechanics, Keaton founded Trybe in 2023 to help high-performing teams and individuals use physical and cognitive tools to thrive.

keatonlynn.com

@keatonlion

Focus on one breath at a time, find your flow, and live with purpose.

Erika exemplifies health in all dimensions: body, mind, relationships, energy, and presence. Her eyes reflect clarity, brightness, and directness — qualities that mirror her approach to medicine.

Her book, *The Nourish Me Kitchen*, is an essential resource that beautifully complements her insights about holistic health and integrating Eastern wisdom into daily wellness practices.

— *Book momma Chandra*

3

The Nuts and Bolts of Chinese Medicine

Dr. Erika Siegel

Chinese medicine, like most holistic modalities, is about restoring harmony. It teaches us to live life in moderation and in accordance with the world around us. Chinese medicine therapies bring balance, seeking to cool what is hot, dry what is damp, move what is stagnant, and replenish what is weak and deficient. These terms, which we do not often use in Western medicine, are rooted in an understanding of the Five Element Theory.

Chinese medicine overview

The five elements — wood, fire, earth, metal, and water — give us the foundation of Chinese medicine theory. Each element has its own associated season, direction, and climate, stage of growth and development, internal organs, body tissue, emotion, aspect of the soul, taste, color, and sound. The five elements reflect a deep understanding of natural law and the interconnectedness of everything, giving us a context in which to describe our observations of the body. And the spark behind the whole machine that governs these five elements is the *Qi* or vital life energy.

Qi (pronounced "chee") is loosely translated as "energy," although there is no exact word for it in conventional Western thought. In the Ayurvedic tradition, a similar concept of flowing energy and life force is called *prana*. In Chinese medicine, Qi is the life force that precedes all matter. It flows throughout the body through channels, or *meridians* and passes to the internal organs. Together with the blood, Qi supplies nourishment to the body and ensures its normal functioning. According to ancient Chinese texts, if blood and Qi fall into disharmony, "a hundred diseases may arise." We are healthy when Qi and blood, the basis of life, are balanced within the body and flow harmoniously. Qi and blood are aspects of *yang* and *yin* respectively.

The art and science of Chinese medicine involve using this philosophy to uncover the exact nature and proper treatment of a person's condition. Diagnosis is based on a detailed account of someone's symptoms and lifestyle, which includes diet, exercise, work, play, emotions, sleep, and sexual habits. Practitioners also evaluate a person's "constitution," or what strengths and weaknesses they were born with. A Chinese medicine intake is very thorough, to say the least, and this deep questioning session is followed by a unique observation of physical signs.

As a Chinese medicine practitioner, I first observe the tongue for its shape, color, and coating, and feels distinct features of the pulse to understand a wealth of information about the body. I observe the skin tone and the smell of the breath and body, and assess the sparkle of spirit emanating from the eyes. I take into account the body posture and feel of the muscles, meridians, and acupuncture points. This thorough method of observing the body represents the vital Chinese medicine concept of the parts reflecting the whole: the microcosm reveals the macrocosm.

From intake to treatment plan

After questioning and observation, this in-depth snapshot of someone's current health informs a detailed and individualized treatment plan. This is very different from symptom based allopathic medicine, in which treatment works to counteract symptoms rather than treat the whole individual.

Here is an example:

Let's say you go to your Western doctor for a headache. Likely the prescription is for a pain reliever, and maybe some suggestions to hydrate better, right?

If you have a headache and go to a Chinese medicine practitioner, you will not just be given a pain-killing herb and then sent on your way. First, the location and quality of the headache will be assessed:

- Pain in the temples reflects a dysfunction in the liver or gallbladder, or perhaps certain foods disturbing those channels.

- A frontal headache is often related to the digestive organs from perhaps hunger, food sensitivities, or constipation.

- Pain in the top of the head reflects a Qi and blood deficiency (dehydration headache is a good example of Qi and blood deficiency).

- A headache coming up from the neck extending like a tight band around the temples is said to be caused by blood and Qi stagnation in the neck and shoulders (tight muscles).

You get the picture: each pattern is different and will be treated differently, taking into account what is happening at the root of the symptom.

As you can see, a treatment plan in this holistic discipline is based on the unique individual, taking multiple factors into account at once. The plan could include any combination of Chinese medicine modalities, including nutrition, herbs, acupuncture, movement, and meditation. These modalities are a way of life when prevention is the cornerstone of your healthcare plan.

Yin and yang explained

Yin and yang underlie all aspects of Chinese philosophy and medicine. They represent the duality within ourselves as well as in the environment around us. We can't have healthy yin without some yang, and vice versa. Allowing them to dance in a dynamic flow is our goal.

Our culture tends to be very *yang,* which is characterized by assertion, productivity, and materialism. Yang's energy is hot and masculine. It is drinking a cup of coffee and going for a run. Having the zest of yang is crucial for activity and progress, but yang will burn up without the balancing nature of yin.

Unfortunately, we tend to undervalue our *yin* need for relaxation, rest, and connecting with the earth. Yin energy feels like a cup of chamomile tea, a big exhale, and a restorative nap. It is feminine and soft. Too much yin, however, leads to inactivity, dampness, and stagnation.

We see yin and yang at play all around us. The introspective yin of winter gives way to the yang spark of spring. The yang of a child excitedly playing is followed by the yin comfort of a nap. A relaxing yin soak in a hot tub invites a revitalizing yang rinse of cold water. Even in its symbol, both yin and yang each have a little bit of their counterpart embedded within. Keep this image in mind as you activate your yang and nourish your yin every day.

Chinese medicine modalities

Nutrition

The interesting thing about Chinese nutrition therapy (as well as Ayurvedic nutrition) is that it looks beyond vitamins, minerals, and macronutrients (carbs, protein, fats), examining instead the *energetic action* of a particular food. A food may be described as warming, cooling, drying, or moistening. Practitioners will consider the therapeutic use of the five flavors — pungent, salty, sour, bitter, and sweet — and a food's action on specific organs.

You may be prescribed food to "nourish the yin" or "clear damp-ness" or told to avoid something like fried foods, which cause the energy in the liver to become agitated. It is quite fascinating indeed.

Recommendations are also based on the season, climate, and an individual's health and digestive power. A Chinese medicine practitioner would be hesitant to recommend smoothies in the middle of a wet winter because the body is already experiencing cold and dampness. Similarly, you're unlikely to see a practitioner recommending a lot of raw food un-less the patient is living in a warm climate and/or has strong digestive capability.

I really appreciate the Chinese teachings on what I will call "digestive hygiene." They emphasize the importance of eating in a slow relaxed fashion, eating during appropriate times of the day, and not putting out the digestive fire with a big glass of water while eating. The ancient texts suggest to "eat breakfast like a king, lunch like a prince, and dinner like a pauper." The spleen and stomach, the organs that transform food into usable nourishment for the body, need to rest during the evening, so dinner should actually be a small meal. In fact, the time of day that the digestive organs get the most blood and energy flow is between 7-11 a.m., just in time to eat like a king.

Acupuncture

One of my favorite aspects of my practice is acupuncture. This ancient technique utilizes small (mostly) painless needles, accessing Qi at specific points. The needles change the flow of energy in the *channel* (energy highway) and its related organ. Qi flows both deep within the body and through channels near the surface. I apply acupuncture needles to the points in each channel where the Qi can be accessed near the surface. A channel may be disturbed and stagnant, which is reflected in pain, stiff-ness, and swelling (think about tight muscles in your neck and shoulders). In such a case, I try to stimulate and move the congestion with my nee-dles. In another case, someone may feel overworked and tired. This is a sign of a deficiency, and my needle "prescription" will focus on rebuilding and nourishing rather than moving. Whatever the treatment, it will have transformative effects on the brain and nervous system.

Something happens on the acupuncture table that I can't quite describe. There is an internal quietness that we, the patient and I, reach together, sometimes through some discomfort, resistance, and even perhaps an emotional release with laughter or tears. I select the individual points for someone and then step away, never knowing what is going to occur as we let the body's intelligence do what it needs to do. I enjoy witnessing and facilitating this, but I also receive benefits from the practice, becoming calm inside as I focus on compassionate care and holding a quiet healing space.

Within minutes of getting on the table, the nervous system switches from the sympathetic (stress) state to the parasympathetic (healing) state. Many of my patients enter a state that they describe as "not quite awake, but not totally asleep." Research shows that during acupuncture, brain waves switch from alpha and beta waves (focused thought and mental chatter) to delta and theta waves (deep sleep and meditation). This may occur with or without the patient falling asleep, but either way, it induces a state of deep relaxation similar to a really good nap or a deep and peaceful meditation session. I stay very humble about the mystery and medicine acupuncture provides.

Herbal medicine

Chinese herbal medicine dates back to 168 BC, with an early collection of over 300 formulas published in 200 AD as the *Shan Han Lun*. Many of these formulas are still used today. There are over 3000 potential products in Chinese herbalism, but most herbalists make use of about 300. They are all called "herbs," but these products actually include leaves, flowers, barks, stems, seeds, and roots, as well as shells and animal and insect parts.

As with food, herbs are evaluated based on their energetics rather than their phytochemicals and active constituents. The temperature of the herb (warming or cooling), the direction of its energy (ascending or descending), and which organ or organ system it affects are described for each herb or herbal combination. For example, the common herb peppermint is described as cooling, pungent, and dry. Its direction is upwards, and it affects the lung meridian and digestive organs. We see this in action when we inhale peppermint oil, and it clears our sinuses or when we drink mint tea to quiet an upset belly.

Movement

Life is all about movement. When there is harmonious flow, there is health. Chinese medicine promotes various movement forms, like Tai chi and Qi gong, to maintain harmonious flow in the body and prevent disease.

Qi gong is a practice meant to elevate and increase awareness of your energy. It utilizes a series of exercises that involve posture, movement, breathing, meditation, and mindfulness. Qi gong, if practiced daily, is truly preventative medicine. There are many different schools and lineages of Qi gong; some focus on the yang, or more forceful movements for physical training, and some are more yin, or gentle in nature, affecting the spiritual body.

Here is a five-minute practice called "Qi gong shaking" that you can do almost anywhere at any time.

Qi gong shaking

Shaking is an excellent way to start or end the day. It's great if you need to literally shake off some weighty thoughts or stuck energy. This practice releases tension by relaxing the muscles and connective tissues. It opens the joints, gently bounces the organs, and detoxifies cells. After just a few minutes of this practice, you may feel refreshed and renewed as your blood and energy noticeably flow with more ease.

- All you need is two to five minutes!

- This is best to do with an empty bladder and belly.

- Ideally, find a natural setting or at least a quiet space.

For the best experience, have someone read these instructions (slowly) to you so you can experience the exercise without having to stop to read them. Alternatively, you can record yourself reading them.

Begin with your feet shoulder-width apart with your knees slightly bent and your feet grounded and heavy. Start the movement from the bottom of your feet by gently bouncing your heels. You do not need to rise up too high, as this may fatigue your calves quickly. Then just bounce and shake in an up-and-down motion, loosely and rhythmically. Lift one foot off the ground at a time as you shake out your ankles and legs. Keep going and shake out those wrists and arms. Keep shaking. Yes, you look strange, but who cares! Go big if you want to or reduce the amplitude of the shake if you prefer. Keep your heels on the ground if you desire but keep bouncing. Breathe freely and fully, letting sounds — weird noises and big sighs — escape from your mouth if that feels right. You can do it! Shake for one minute or several minutes.

Return to stillness slowly by making the motions smaller and smaller until they are physically imperceptible. Feel your energy ground back into your feet. Then be still for a minute and feel the continuing internal vibrations. You will feel warm, tingly, and open, with increased blood and Qi flow. What you are feeling is QI MOVING. Doesn't that feel good?! When Qi is moving freely, your mind and body will feel more in the flow.

Massage

Massage is like Qi gong being done to you by someone else. Oriental massage includes Shiatsu, Tuina, acupressure, and a number of additional techniques focusing on the meridians and body as a whole, all facilitating smooth movement of the Qi. Like all Chinese modalities, the goal of massage is to strengthen areas that are weak and disperse areas that are blocked.

Bodywork extends beyond the physical body, encouraging emotional states to come up to the surface and disperse rather than creating stagnation and pain in the inner world of the body. The goal of the Chinese medicine practitioner (and hopefully all practitioners!) is to touch the body with loving kindness and compassion. This quality of touch is in many ways as therapeutic as the physical massage action itself.

Massage is something most of us can do for our loved ones. It can be especially beneficial for children. I recommend massaging children frequently, especially when they are ill or upset. When kids are acting wild and totally out of sorts, that is the time when they need to feel their bodies the most, and most kids will calm right down for some rubbing from their beloved adult. We have gotten through some hard times with our kids by choosing a hand or foot massage over a timeout (it makes me feel better too, especially when I am at my wits' end). I can always tell when my older son is feeling a bit tender because he will ask me for a little massage at bedtime. Don't be held back by thinking you need to massage in a certain way; just get a little oil (jojoba or coconut oil works great) and go to it.

I am particularly fond of using tools (like flat stones, jade, or even the side of a metal spoon) to massage the skin in a technique called gua sha. Gua sha is also known as scraping or spooning. In chiropractic medicine, it has evolved into the "Graston technique," which is a little different. These instrument-assisted massages can be done by yourself (like the popular facial techniques to reduce puffiness and wrinkles) or by someone else to large or small swaths of the body. Gua means "scrape" and sha means "petechiae" or "sand". The petechiae are reddish-purple spots that look like hickeys, which you might also see in "cupping" (which I also love!). They tell you that you are moving some serious Qi! Think of gua sha as an immediate way to get blood flowing, which of course means that it promotes healing.

Gua sha began as a full-body treatment but can be used effectively on specific areas. I will often work someone's entire back with long firm strokes for about 5-10 minutes, which powerfully invigorates blood flow and detoxifies their entire body. In fact, one patient said she sweated profusely for 12 hours after her treatment while her body continued to release toxins. Many others report feeling completely renewed after receiving that treatment.

Gua sha is one of my favorite tools for boosting children's immune systems when they are feeling a little crummy- and it's so easy for anyone to perform (I massage some carrier oil with a few drops of eucalyptus oil onto the chest and back and scrape from the sternum out, and from the spine out and down). Gua sha home-facial techniques have recently become very popular, which is pretty cool. You can use those same tools and techniques anywhere on the body for muscle tension and fascial adhesions. Gua sha is simple and effective, and while it may cause some temporary discomfort and bruising (if you really go for it), the discomfort will go away quickly, restoring the tissue and the areas beneath to better balance.

Meditation

Chinese medicine teaches that it is most important to nourish the spirit, and it is of secondary importance to nourish the body. The spirit, also called the *Shen,* should be "pure and tranquil" for lasting health and vitality. There are forms of meditation and mindfulness in almost every culture; the most significant Chinese meditation practices have Taoist and Buddhist influences. The main goal of meditation is to quiet the mind in order to experience stillness and relaxation. This is done regularly by focusing on posture, breathing, and perhaps a mantra (a repeated prayer or saying).

A commitment to meditation is obviously a huge challenge for many of us. Taking on a new daily practice can feel totally overwhelming and honestly not worth the time. Besides, it is so hard to just sit still! But the reality is that mindfulness practice enhances every area of our health, and meditation and visualization can actually reverse disease. For instance, high blood pressure, often a "silent killer" contributing to heart attacks and stroke, can be better balanced with both prayer and meditation. That's some powerful medicine available to all.

Key takeaways to implement

✳ Balance the yin and yang

Remember that every exhale needs an inhale — try to spend your time with this awareness of daily balance. Try to weave in restorative breaks into a busy day as well as challenge yourself (both mentally and physically) if your tendency is to sink too much into comfort zones that are perhaps a bit too comfortable.

✳ Practice digestive hygiene

Before eating, take a few breaths, and bring your attention to this very moment with mindfulness and intention. This allows the digestive fire to build. Enjoy your food slowly and don't put out that fire with a big glass of water while eating. Remember, the ancient texts suggest to "Eat breakfast like a king, lunch like a prince, and dinner like a pauper." And I will add that after dinner, you don't need any more food to fuel the day.

✳ Move your body everyday

In big and small ways. Movement is life — it will circulate QI and blood which brings nutrition in and waste out. Try the simple Qi gong exercise above for a really efficient movement practice.

✳ Massage

Others and yourself! Try Gua sha tools for really moving that fascia and restoring proper qi flow. You can find many options online.

✳ Find a practitioner

If after reading this, you are ready to find a Chinese medicine practitioner, check: www.nccaom.org and when choosing a Chinese medicine practitioner, it is best to find someone with a master's or doctorate in oriental medicine (MSOM, DAOM) instead of someone who learned acupuncture over a weekend course (these are often available to chiropractors, osteopaths, and medical doctors).

About the author

Dr. Erika Siegel is a naturopathic physician, acupuncturist, educator, and mom: by nature, a juggler of life's abundance. She's been practicing functional, integrative medicine for over 20 years, offering whole-bodied health care and inspiration to thrive. Dr. Siegel continuously expands her knowledge of therapies from around the globe to support others in maintaining the balance of mind, body, and spirit.

Her two-volume book set, *The Nourish Me Kitchen*, combines a first-of-its-kind functional medicine reference book along with a stunning wholesome-foods cookbook. Through these books you get an inside view of Dr. Siegel's practical knowledge and time-tested expertise — backed by peer-reviewed research — empowering you to support and heal yourself with food, medicine, home remedies, herbs, and self-care.

Discover the foundations of your personal wellness and illuminate the mysteries of how your body works through this integrative, East-meets-West field guide for living vibrantly and aging gracefully. You can learn more about Chinese and Naturopathic functional medicine and her work at:

www.nourishme.com

Erin's naturopathic perspective on labs — a viewpoint that differs significantly from conventional medicine — is one I highly recommend. Having a naturopathic doctor review your bloodwork can enlighten you to see patterns and possibilities that standard analysis likely misses.

Her natural remedies and her hydrotherapy approaches greatly help my family and will help your family's health too.

— *Book momma Chandra*

4

Naturopathic Medicine from Womb to Wisdom Years

Erin Frances Sharman, ND

Each human is born with a certain amount of potential. In my field of work, I describe it as vitality. How much vitality do you have for the world? How much capacity do you possess to defend and restore your physical, emotional, and mental body each day after it encounters infections, environmental toxins, stressors, emotions, intake of food and air, physical activity — daily life. Some people are given the short end of the stick in this matter, and some are rather gifted and are given a huge capacity. As a Naturopathic doctor (ND), my goal is to holistically increase each person's capacity for vitality so that they can realize their unique potential.

By the end of this chapter, it is my utmost wish that you walk away with an understanding that there are many, many options for health and healing and that each person has a HUGE potential to impact their health through their everyday diet and lifestyle.

If you optimize your health, during the beginning stages of disease you will have a better shot at overcoming your disease. Or even a step further — if you optimize your health before conception, you can radically increase the vital capacity and the potential of your child before they are even born.

First, I want to share the differences between regular Western medicine and the type of holistic medicine I practice — Naturopathic medicine. Second, I'll offer holistic solutions you may not know about yet.

Naturopathic medicine is a very different paradigm; most individuals who see me for the first time are not used to having a physician who wants to get so nuanced and engaged with their health. The Western medical world tends to look at the body as a state of health or of disease with very little in between.

The four differences: Labs, depth, pharmaceuticals, and prevention

Difference number one: Labs

NDs look at lab values differently than typical MDs. A MD makes sure that your labs are within the normal lab values. If your result is above the standard range, then this is cause for investigation or treatment. If your labs are in the normal range but just about to be out of range, then typically, the advice is to come back in six months to a year and retest.

However, when I look at labs, I want to see the lab values be *optimal.* This is a much narrower range and if the lab values are out of the optimal, then I encourage the individual to change something *now* in their life so that the numbers will ideally return to an optimal range.

Difference number two: Depth

Depth of questioning with Naturopathic medicine differs from traditional Western medicine. It's not good enough to know that you have a regular bowel movement — I want to know the timing, the consistency, the quality, and other signs of your digestion. Do you burp? Do you have gas and boating? Do you have stomach pain? Does your stool have undigested food?

Difference number three: Pharmaceuticals

Western doctors offer pharmaceutical interventions often without considering or informing you of the cost on your body. It is not uncommon for my patients to express remorse after taking pharmaceutical medications. I often hear, "No one ever told me that this could happen."

For example, oral contraceptives (birth control pills) are given without explanation of long-term effects. Studies[1] have shown that long-term use of oral contraceptives can cause consistent elevations of a hormone called sex hormone binding globulin (SHBG) that persists even after a woman discontinues the pill. This long-term elevation can cause decreased production of sex hormones (namely testosterone and estrogen) and have long-term effects on arousal, muscle mass, fertility, and overall aging. Oral contraceptives definitely have a purpose and place in this world; however, it is important that women be aware of the many other options that are available and weigh the benefits and risks associated with each treatment.

Difference four: Prevention

One of the most important lessons I've learned, and one that most of us unfortunately need to learn the hard way, is that prevention truly is key. As parents, our job is to notice the slight changes in our child's mood and physical body when it shifts to a state of stress or decreased functioning and then to help restore their body to a state of vitality. This is a full-time job! But it also prevents children from getting so sick that they need more aggressive medical intervention. I always recommend cleaning up the child's diet and sleep habits immediately when a parent notices any signs or symptoms of illness. Natural therapies, like diet and sleep, have so much power to alter the course of an illness. These therapies do take time and effort, but they also have a much superior result when started at the onset of an illness rather than once the illness has developed.

Holistic toolbox

One of the most beautiful parts of Naturopathic medicine is that NDs have a HUGE toolbox to use; meaning we can tailor the treatment plan to each patient's likes and dislikes. For example, some patients won't take capsules, others cannot tolerate alcohol-based preparations, and others want to do everything they can with diet and lifestyle before they take any sort of supplements. I love finding a protocol that exactly fits the person I am working with. If I can make the treatment plan palatable and easy for the patient to adhere to then it is a win-win situation!

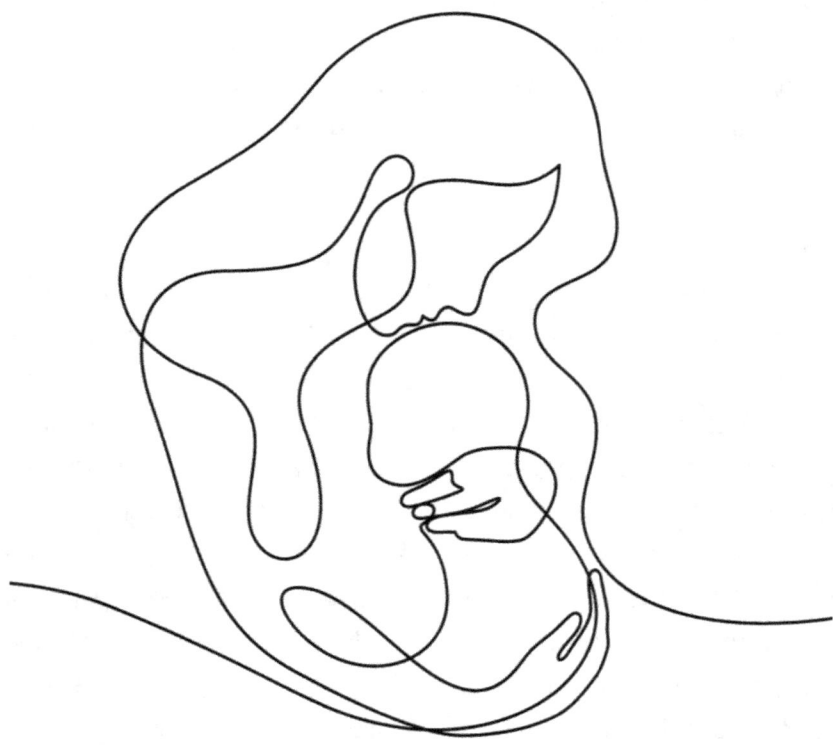

Optimization during conception and childhood

When you set intentions and plan for conception, you can actualize the most potential. I love working with both women and men to optimize their well-being before conception, and I encourage them to also optimize their emotional and spiritual well-being so that when the baby is conceived, the genetic and emotional being that forms in that moment is at its maximal state.

Obviously, not everyone can prepare in such a planned and predetermined way. Luckily, there is still great room for improvement during a child's or infant's early life. I feel especially passionate about helping caretakers and their children navigate all of the health issues that arise in the first few years of life.

Holistic and preventative medicine shines here! For example, in my decade-plus of being a physician, I have never had to give a child antibiotics for an ear infection. I've found that ear infections are fairly easy to control with the use of dietary changes, herbal and physical stimulation of the immune system, and homeopathy. The same goes for childhood eczema and common digestive issues found in childhood, like constipation, diarrhea, and reflux.

I'll never forget this woman who came to see the busy primary care clinic setting I was working at. She had a four-month-old daughter that had been put on acid blockers for reflux. The mother had very little knowledge about nutrition and had not been given any other options to treat her daughter's digestive discomfort. We made a simple suggestion to try removing dairy from mom's diet as the daughter was 100 percent breastfed, and we gave her a homeopathic medication to be taken twice daily. The mom was able to immediately discontinue the acid-blocking medication, and her baby no longer suffered from reflux/digestive issues and, in turn, was a happier, more content baby.

One of my favorite techniques is using hydrotherapy or water to help stimulate the immune system. The physical push and pull of alternating hot and cold deliver something that oral medication cannot: a direct therapeutic intervention enhancing the function of an area of the body. Here is an example of one of my favorite hydrotherapy treatments, often referred to as constitutional hydrotherapy.

Hydrotherapy story

During spring break, of course all three of my kiddos got high fevers. We were traveling and staying in a rural cabin in the Sierras. I had no access to the normal array of natural medicines I would typically be shoving down their throats every couple of hours. The first night, I felt helpless and sorry for myself and stayed up way too late worrying about my predicament. The next morning, I kicked myself into action. Enough was enough. I needed to get these kids better. What could I do for them with the limited supplies at hand? Then I remembered hydrotherapy.

Maybe it's because we are in a culture that is so oriented to "pill-popping," but for some reason, I constantly have to remind myself that hydrotherapy is truly one of the most effective methods we can use to help our bodies naturally boost the immune system to find health and balance.

I got out a bunch of hand towels, a beach towel for each kid, and two large pots filled with the hottest and coldest water the faucet would deliver — the cold was very mountain cold. Then I got to work.

I started by putting each kid faceup in their bed on top of a beach towel, simply to make sure the bed stayed dry. I then placed a well wrung, folded in half, hot hand towel over their belly and chest. I covered them each with a blanket and waited three minutes. Then, I refreshed the hot towel with a new one for two more minutes. While waiting for the two minutes to be up, I readied the cold hand towel (again folded in half and well-wrung). I did a final hot refresh for one minute; each time, making sure to recover with the blanket, and then swapped the hot towel out for the cold towel, which sat for 10 minutes.

Phew! I was halfway done. All I had left was to repeat the above with the child lying on their belly and the folded towel covering their shoulders down to their lower back.

By the time I finished the treatment, I had a quiet cabin of sleeping children.

An added benefit to doing this treatment is that your patient usually falls asleep, AND it is a great way to trick your kids into being quiet and staying in their beds. I repeated the treatment three times that day and two times the following day. I felt empowered and my kids were getting better.

We talk a lot about magic in my household right now, my kids are slightly obsessed with magic.

If magic is found in this world, it certainly exists in hydrotherapy!

I particularly love treating children because they generally respond very favorably and quickly to Naturopathic treatments. The above examples are just a small window into the value of using diet and lifestyle therapies to quickly and effectively change a child's health for the better. I've seen dramatic shifts in children's health when caretakers are coached in relevant diet and lifestyle changes. I hope you find the courage and motivation to try some!

A small price to pay with PHRT

As a woman, you can reach a whole new set of aging potential by utilizing bio-identical hormone therapy. You can stave off many declines that come with menopause with a rhythmic bio-identical hormone treatment alternative called Physiologic Hormone Restoration Therapy (PHRT). It is a new type of hormone therapy that is nuanced enough to recreate the highs and lows of estrogen and progesterone that are seen in a woman during their reproductive prime. PHRT is one of the most novel women's health protocols I know of and the one I plan to use myself. I plan to have my period into my 80s!

The typical hormone regimen offered to women when menopausal symptoms arise is commonly static hormone therapy with the same low dose of estrogen and progesterone taken daily. This dosing regimen is not based on optimizing a woman's hormones or mimicking any natural process of the body - it is simply an easily administered strategy that thinks of progesterone only as a way to balance the effects of estrogen on the uterine lining.

This typical approach lacks awareness and consideration of progesterone's incredibly potent processes in the body. It neglects the nuanced interplay between the peaks of estrogen and progesterone during the first and second half of a woman's typical cycle. This nuance is integral to turning on and off hundreds of genes that help regulate function in the body.

There can be some benefit in using static hormone therapy as it does help relieve some of the typical symptoms associated with menopause. But the static Western approach is the same low dose every day. Whereas the PHRT approach is far more nuanced in timing and dosage which has the vital effect of preventing typical menopausal caused diseases and decline like dementia, heart disease, osteoporosis, changes in the skin, and low libido.

The beauty of PHRT is that it can restore and stave off the above diseases and prevent changes like typical skin decline and low libido that take place in menopause after peak levels of estrogen and progesterone drop.

The protocol changes dramatically depending on what day of the cycle you are on and requires different applications of bio-identical creams twice daily. Because the protocol mimics the highs and lows of a cycling female in her hormonal prime — a menstrual cycle is part of the deal.

I often hear, "Are you crazy?" And I get it. At first, this is a major turn-off to many women. However, once all of the benefits are understood (literally anti-aging in all systems of the body), most realize that a menstrual cycle is a small price to pay.

When dosed correctly, PHRT results in a *polite* menstrual cycle void of heavy bleeding, aches, and pains. I recommend the website womenshormonenetwork.org to anyone who is interested in this protocol — it is an amazing resource for articles and facts about the various types of HRT available and the benefits and risks associated with each protocol.

Natural anti-aging therapies

It is normal to want to look beautiful and retain youthful characteristics as long as possible — this is why the MedSpa industry has exploded with high demand for anti-aging options like Botox and fillers. When it comes to a Naturopathic perspective, it is known that fillers are toxins being injected into areas of the body to paralyze them and thus create the look of youth. There are downstream risks involved with fillers — permanent distortion in facial expressions, scarring, and allergic reactions, to name a few.

I have found microneedling and PRP to be a powerful, natural and effective tool to help stave off the aging process without the downstream risks.

Microneedling

Microneedling is a medical procedure that creates thousands of micro punctures in the skin. The process triggers an inflammatory response, which in turn activates blood flow and initiates the creation of new cells. These new cells are rich in collagen and elastin, which improve the elasticity, thickness, and youth of the skin. Microneedling can be a standalone treatment or can be combined with platelet rich plasma.

Platelet rich plasma (PRP)

Platelet rich plasma (PRP) is a concentrated solution derived from your own blood. After a simple blood draw is performed, the blood is spun in a specialized centrifuge. This is necessary to separate and concentrate the platelet rich portion of the blood from the remainder of the blood.

Platelets are rich in growth factors and play a vital role in healing and tissue regeneration. PRP is used in many areas of medicine that require the healing of injured or aging tissues. It can be used to stimulate hair growth, help heal tendons and ligaments, as well as shorten the healing time of injuries.

PRP is a storage house of growth factors that stimulate tissue regeneration and cell reproduction. Because PRP is from the patient's own blood (via a simple blood draw), it is safe and highly individualized.

When microneedling is combined with PRP, the plasma is applied to the skin before and after the microneedling treatment. The application before the treatment allows the plasma to penetrate the layers of the skin and increase the remodeling and regeneration of the skin.

In conjunction with microneedling, PRP effectively treats acne or surgical scars, wrinkles, fine lines, uneven skin texture, irregularities, and stretch marks, and as a stand-alone treatment, PRP can help restore a thicker and fuller head of hair.

I call PRP for hair restoration a magic wand! I think it is amazing that this treatment combines such minimal recovery time and little to no side effects with positive results.

My doctor's orders to you reader

I urge you to recognize the profound impact you can have on your life by dedicating time, energy, and awareness to optimizing your health and that of your family. The choices you make, from treatment options to early intervention, shape the trajectory of your well-being.

Naturopathic medicine offers a robust toolkit of options that extends far beyond the boundaries of traditional Western medicine. It's not merely about managing illness; it's about proactively enhancing your quality of life — your vital capacity.

Embrace the holistic options, strive for optimal health, and feel your best.

Note

[1] Panzer, C., Wise, S., Fantini, G., et al. (2006). Impact of oral contraceptives on sex hormone-binding globulin and androgen levels: A retrospective study in women with sexual dysfunction. *The Journal of Sexual Medicine*, 3(1), 104–113. https://doi.org/10.1111/j.1743-6109.2005.00198.x

Key takeaways to implement

* Use hydrotherapy first — before using antibiotics next time you or a loved one is feverish. Go to my blog post on hydrotherapy https://www.theremedymartinez.com/blog/hydrotherapy for instructions.

* Get to know your options for your health. Invest in natural anti-aging options locally. I am located in Martinez, California and service the general bay area.

* Get HRT hormone support in your 40s — don't wait until you have symptoms. PRHT resource: womenshormonenetwork.org.

* Order your labs with your Western doctor and have me or another ND look at your labs through an optimizing lens. You can book a consult with me here: https://www.drerinsharman.com/workwithus

* Remember there are options! Come see me or another ND if you aren't feeling well and your regular doctor says you are fine!

About the author

Dr. Sharman is passionate about supporting individuals in their journey to regain the utmost health and happiness.

Dr. Erin Sharman earned her Naturopathic Doctorate from the National University of Natural Medicine. After graduating, she completed a 2-year certified post-doctoral residency with *A Family Healing Center*, emphasizing primary care, pediatrics, and pain management. As a family practitioner, she has extensive training in pediatrics, women's health, pain management, cardiovascular disease, nutrition counseling, gastrointestinal disease, thyroid management, and hormone balancing. Her latest endeavor is natural anti-aging techniques.

During her studies, Dr. Sharman completed a two-year clinical mentorship in women's health under the direction of Dr. Kimberly Windstar and a six—month internship focusing on chronic disease management and biotherapeutic drainage with Dr. Dickson Thom. She has additional training in Ayurvedic medicine and has a certification in Ayurvedic Herbalism. Dr. Sharman believes strongly in the holistic approach to medicine, integrating nutritional and lifestyle counseling, herbal medicine, and homeopathy to provide individualized patient-centered care.

When she is not practicing medicine, Dr. Sharman is a mother of three, farmhand, dancer, musician, and explorer.

drerinsharman.com

"Julie is a national asset," said one of the many people I've referred to her. When she chose this chapter topic, I was initially surprised. She explained, "I kept asking myself: what is the one most important thing that will help people step into their potential? This is it."

Her insight is compelling — if our cells aren't functioning optimally, our entire system struggles.

—*Book Momma Chandra*

5

The Core Fix for Starving Cells: Trace Minerals and Cell Salts

Julie North

As a lifelong medium and a Medical Intuitive for more than 30 years, I've come to understand a tremendous amount about the human experience and what impacts both the experience *and* our potential as individuals.

My work has me regularly delving into the details of a person's physical and non-physical well-being, struggles, and solutions. Year after year, I continue to see a steady stream of people who are all suffering physically, mentally, emotionally, energetically, and spiritually. Most people can't seem to figure out why they're struggling to maintain a balanced baseline of wellness across the board. They all *want* to be better but they're at a loss for why they're stuck. They're desperate to find a path that brings them back into balance. Thriving would be ideal, but it seems like such an insurmountable task given where they currently find themselves. Regardless of the wide and varied experiences and situations that bring people to my work, there is an extremely common fundamental issue that about 90 percent of them share.

Most of the people I come across in the Medical Intuitive readings that I do for individuals, and in the world at large, are missing the fundamental keys to not only their wellness but to expanding and securing their personal potential. By the time people make their way to me, they've often been through multitudes of doctors, specialists, and therapists, done rigorous research of their own, and tried untold numbers of healing modalities, all to find themselves plateaued on their path for unknown reasons. They are frequently unable to maintain what they have already achieved, let alone reach their higher goals. Efforts to build upon their current state have proven insurmountable for reasons they cannot figure out. They're frustrated, and their care professionals are perplexed. Because the cause is unknown, the core issue is not resolved. The path forward is typically one of cascading new issues and chasing symptoms. It's a cycle that leaves most people exhausted, disheartened, and slowly getting worse.

Making your efforts effective

Then there is almost everyone else. Maybe they're not in survival mode but nonetheless somehow "stuck" in their lives. They're existing but not "living." They lack emotional well-being and good mental health and feel somehow disconnected from themselves, others, and their energy or spiritual world, regardless of what they call it. They aren't technically sick, but they aren't at their best, either. They often express low energy, lack of joy, and a general apathy toward life. Despite "doing all the things" they can't seem to get any tangible forward movement. They cannot get over their unknown hurdle and *live* their life to the fullest. Keenly aware that they could be *so much more* than who and how they are currently living, they just can't break through. They may even have healthy diets, exercise regularly, meditate, get bodywork or energy work, and have a regular spiritual practice, all to little or no avail. Most people I talk to these days are exhausted from making marginal headway, only to see their progress backslide after a short time. They're depressed, sometimes anxious, losing hope, exhausted, and at their wit's end. Though their struggles may not be related to physical ailments, these people usually lack the exact same foundational components that has others gravely unwell.

To be fair, most people are often doing their best, with the information that they have, to heal their body, mind, spirit, or energetic system. So why do they not reach their healthiest potential? It begets a laundry list of common questions and complaints. Why did I start getting better and then falter? Why aren't my treatments and medications working? Why can't I stay positive? I am doing all the right things and have great relationships in my life, but I just don't feel *happy*. I meditate and get energy work, but I can't seem to stay in balance. I eat all organic food and work out, but I don't have any energy. I just feel "off" and sluggish. Whether physical, mental, emotional, or energetic, an unseen hurdle links them all, and almost no one talks about it.

Modern medicine and mental healthcare are truly a miracle. We can all attest to the advancements they have made in saving and extending lives, as well as improving the quality of those lives. There simply is no replacement for much of what allopathic medicine can now do for a person. Yet somehow, there seems to be a gap in understanding that undermines much of their efforts. What is it that lies at the very core of our *being, which affects each system independently, as well as how they interact with each other? *Being is to denote your physical body and your energetic body in their wholeness.

There could be as many unique reasons as there are unique people, of course. But one thing they all have in common is a physical body and a non-physical body, working in conjunction with one another to comprise the human experience. Billions of individuals with different bodies, different soul paths, different emotional experiences, different teachings, and beliefs... and yet they all share a foundational system of a physical body, energetic body, and the connecting aspects between them. With these many variables, what could possibly serve them all? What not only helps us survive but opens us up to a wide and wondrous world of possibilities and potential? What if you could help heal the two foundational components that affect both the physical *and* the energetic body at the same time? You can, and it's so easy that it hardly seems capable of being the fundamental miracle that it usually is. It's simple for certain, but there is no workaround for meeting this need. As I've mentioned, it's foundational. There is no shortcut, but it is so easy it doesn't really need one.

The fundamental miracle

Thirty-plus years as a medical medium has shown me that a deficiency in trace minerals *and* the twelve essential cell salts is the epidemic problem that undermines the well-being of all these systems. Thousands of people I have worked with have reported previously unattainable healing and truly life-changing results from addressing this little-known issue. Doctors I've worked with have sometimes validated these deficiencies later through rare cellular testing or hair analysis reports, as well as reporting on patient health improvements once supplemented. Mental health practitioners have relayed drastic changes for themselves and their patients. Previously unsuccessful strategies for healing began working more effectively and were better sustained once remineralization of these trace minerals began. Energy-sensitive people, healers, and practitioners also report a greater ability to manage their own energy. They have improved clarity, better intuition, and overall better energetic balance after addressing these deficiencies. These drastic improvements allow people to expand and achieve their potential healing and wellness, even when all the other avenues they'd explored had faltered. Why?

The core fix

Trace minerals and cell salts are two separate classifications and must be addressed separately. Your body requires both to operate properly on *any* level. While most of us are aware we need nutrition for a healthy system, our knowledge of exactly what nutrition we need is limited to what our science has known and shared with us. Most of us have a limited awareness of basic vitamins and common minerals, functions, and needs. Because so little has been known about trace minerals in the health care and science world, most people wouldn't have any idea that these even existed, let alone how they are being impacted by the lack of them. Even now, there are very few studies detailing these important elements.

Understanding the physical and non-physical human body

Before we jump into the core fix, it's helpful to have a better understanding of the human body. There are two primary components of a human being: their physical aspect and their non-physical aspect. These two parts require each other for the baseline experience as a human being. Each has needs specifically related to their respective parts and a couple that they directly share. It is these fundamental shared pieces that have, in my opinion, the most profound impact on the human being and the human experience at such a foundational level. If these shared potentiators are lacking, all other efforts see minimized improvements, if any. Without these rarely known or discussed building blocks in place, the entire system and experience is not only incapable of proper basic function but cannot even consider expanding or achieving its potential.

Most of us can easily understand that if we want the physical body to survive, we need to meet very basic requirements for food (nutrition) and water. If, however, we want to reach our potential, to have the endurance to run a marathon, be able to climb mountains without getting winded, or live longer with fewer health issues, we need to have more nutritious food and cleaner water, both with greater frequency. Most of us have personal firsthand experience with this in our own lives. The healthier we are, the more we can physically do and endure.

The non-physical body, however, is less universally agreed upon in name and function. This non-physical aspect may be called the Soul or the Energy Body, amongst other names, and serves for most people to define or encapsulate those areas of a human experience that do not have a solid form. These things might be called energy, intuition, emotion, thoughts, beliefs, kundalini, or other names, depending on your knowledge or belief pattern. For the sake of our conversation here, we will call this non-physical half of the human experience the "energy body."

Chronic compensation

Humans are resilient beings with an amazing capacity to compensate for a lack, an injury, or a trauma until a resolution can happen. Compensation is meant to be a temporary work-around, though, and not the standard of operation. Any deficiency or injury that goes on too long creates a domino effect of issues. These subsequent issues are part of that compensation chain, but their symptoms often appear unrelated to the original problem. This leaves people baffled as to the cause of these down-the-line symptoms or issues. The same is true for trace mineral and cell salt deficiencies, as you will see later in this chapter.

Physical body

The more obvious and familiar compensating effects within each system are easily understood. If we injure our shoulder and it doesn't heal properly, we'd rightly assume that our long-term pain is the result. We might even accurately link our subsequent arm numbness to that same injury if we can realize it came on as our shoulder was wounded, healing or closely thereafter. But what if, a year later, you ended up with lower back pain and a sore hip? Unless you have intimate knowledge of how the fascia in the body is connected, as well as how it compensates, you'd likely think this was an entirely new issue and try to treat it as such. You might get regular massages on the lower back and hip that would briefly alleviate the pain, but the relief wouldn't last. Only once the locked tissues of the shoulder were released would the lower-back work be effective. Why? Because the chain of tightening still originates at the shoulder, even if you can't feel that anymore. This, in turn, creates a chain of pulling that eventually pulls on an entirely different part of your body. That core problem in the shoulder will *keep* causing issues elsewhere until it is addressed. The body's organs are like the gears in a watch, all calibrated to one another. When one organ system struggles, another may falter due to this breakdown in calibration and overall function.

Non-physical body

Energetic body compensation isn't any different. Whether it's emotional, mental, spiritual, or energetic, consistently unhealthy systems will eventually result in additional illness and issues elsewhere. For example, a single unhealed emotional trauma can cause seemingly unrelated dysfunctional processing of information, even in unrelated areas of thought. Down the line, this unresolved issue can create additional emotional imbalances, a distortion of "reality," disproportionate responses, and difficulty regulating one's survival wiring.

Less is commonly known about the basic needs of the energy body, though much speculation exists. What most of us, however, subscribe to is the idea that we indeed have some form of energy body and that it somehow interacts with, or through, the physical form. Much like the more subtle and intricate workings of the physical form, we rarely know what is happening in the energetic body or what it needs. We may be aware of the symptoms a dysregulated system creates but we don't know exactly how to fix it. There are a growing number of modalities available today to help clear and heal the energetic body, such as reiki, acupuncture, sound healing, and more. These healing tools will obviously not work as well if they are applied to a system that lacks foundational functionality. Just like traditional bodywork, the positive effects of energy work are often short-lived.

The web of core needs

These two systems do not operate independently of one another either. They are intrinsically tied together, informing each other of their status and impacting each other's potential — *your potential*. It is widely known and accepted that the physical body's health or illness has a direct impact on non-physical health. This is evidenced by how nutritional deficiencies negatively impact a person's mood and emotional health. Studies have even shown that poor nutrition is closely linked to increased acts of crime. The converse is also widely accepted. The energetic body's health or dysfunction has just as great an impact on the physical system. This is readily seen in the effects stress has on the physical body, how someone can literally die of a broken heart, and how continued mental distress compromises the immune system. If a person's issue truly is only located in *one* of these bodies, then a specific modality for that body will likely work. If, however, there is a breakdown in the core needs that these two bodies share, then healing does not happen as hoped. This is the case for almost everyone in the developed world.

The twelve essential cell salts and trace minerals are at the very foundation of both bodies, as well as the system that connects them. Without these underlying needs met, neither system is stable or fully functional. Your very potential, on every conceivable front, is therefore directly tied to whether you have or do not have healthy levels of these obscure minerals and salts in your system.

Think of it as if you were building your home. Your body IS your home, after all, making this is an excellent metaphor for conveying this idea. You only get to build this *one* home. Your whole life is lived in this single home. You can make repairs, remodel it, expand it, or demolish parts as your needs adjust, but whatever you want to do in your life, it's all taking place in this one and only home. Before you can build the bedrooms, bathrooms, kitchen, and living spaces that you're going to be in all the time, celebrating, recharging, and creating amazing ideas, you must build the *foundation*. That foundation is what *everything else* rests upon. If the foundation is built poorly, your home suffers. You'd need to do some repair work to that foundation, or the home will consistently degrade until the walls crack, the floor becomes unsafe, and the roof starts falling in. The wall will just keep cracking, no matter how many times you patch it unless you fix the foundation. Trace minerals and cell salts *are* the foundation of your home; your body and your energy systems.

The science or lack of

Trace minerals are not widely studied or understood by most science or health professionals. They are called "trace minerals" mainly for two reasons. They typically only occur in our food in tiny or "trace" amounts, and the body only needs most of them in a similar trace amount. Modern science isn't even completely aligned with which minerals they'd like to classify as trace minerals for the body. Some studies say there are eight, some say around twenty, and some much, much more. Current science classifies only a few of these trace minerals as "essential" and the rest are labeled as either "essential but uncertain" or "non-essential" simply because they haven't yet determined their exact function in the system. My experience and the testimonials of countless others I've worked with clearly suggest to me that taking a trace mineral compound that contains at least seventy trace minerals, is crucial to achieving the monumental impact most people are seeking.

Trace minerals used to be in the soil, so they were in all our food. In most industrialized countries, the soil has been depleted, and therefore the food is depleted. Even organic produce is often grown in soil that has been mass-farmed and has not yet recovered. It's better than conventionally grown food, but there is no guarantee that all of these barely known minerals have repopulated that soil.

Each individual trace mineral has at least one very specific function in our body. Without that mineral, the body must try and compensate. Selenium, for example, is the trace mineral that allows our thyroid to pick up the iodine it needs to work properly. Without an adequate selenium load in our system, the iodine simply cannot be utilized, and the thyroid is dysfunctional. The thyroid is like the orchestra conductor of the body. In many ways, it keeps all the organ systems working together. If you've ever heard the chaos of an orchestra warming up, with everyone playing their own instruments and tunes, you can imagine what the body does when the thyroid isn't working properly, all because it doesn't have the trace amount of selenium that it needs. This is a single example of just *one* of the things selenium does. When you begin to account for the more than seventy trace minerals needed and all that they impact, you begin to see the downward spiral that can happen. If you or your care providers are not aware of these mineral needs, then the likely path of resolution will be more like patching the cracked wall in a house that actually needs the foundation addressed. The issues will resurface and continue as well as domino into additional problems that get chased in the same less effective manner.

Cellular communication

I have learned through my work, that as a conglomerate, trace minerals do two additional and critical things. The first is where they really impact the energy of the body *and* the communication between the physical and energetic systems. Trace minerals seem to be at the core of proper cell-to-cell communication. Since your entire being is literally built on cell-to-cell communication, the overall deficiency negatively impacts the system's ability to transfer information throughout the system. If your body sends a signal that it needs an immune system response some-where, that signal may not get to its intended target. If it does manage to arrive, the subsequent signal sent out to accomplish the task may not arrive. Your body may have had all that it needed to resolve the issue, but it just didn't get the message. Every muscle movement of your body, every hormone-balancing request, and everything that the body does requires this cell-to-cell communication to work efficiently.

Additionally, every feeling and thought, the magnetic resonance of your heart, and how those feelings and thoughts inform the physical sys-tem all rely on this exact same signaling system to move energy throughout your being. Our emotions run *through* the physical system. This is how trauma can get stuck in the body. The system needs these trace minerals to be able to effectively move energy *through* the system. This is also why almost everyone has a similar response to hearing some-thing sad, their hands go to cover their heart. There's no outside physical object propelling toward our chest that our hands need to block. The energy of sadness runs through the system, and we *feel it* physically in the heart, causing another signal that has our hands protect or offer support to the affected area. There are many such examples of common physical responses to a non-physical impetus. Energy moves *through* the same system and informs the body. Thousands upon thousands of signals are sent within your system every day. Millions maybe. So how would you heal, be well, or endeavor to reach your potential when the most basic of systems that you'd need to achieve this isn't working properly?

Cellular nutrition

The second area that trace minerals affect is the cell's ability to uptake nutrition. On the cell wall are receptors. When the cell needs a nutrient, it tells those receptors. They then must look for that nutrient, grab it, and pull it in through the cell wall. If the cell itself is not properly mineralized, any part of that process can fail. You could get your blood tested, and the results could show that you have "all" the needed nutrition in your blood. The inference from these common tests is that if the nutrition is in your blood, then it's getting to your cells. It simply isn't true. You can have amazing nutritional density in your blood, and your cells are starving. I see it all the time. Only a cellular test can tell you what your cells are up-taking, and even that test will only show for those specific types of cells. If they scrape your calf for the test, that won't necessarily tell you if your liver is absorbing what it needs. It's still more reliable than a blood test, but it's often expensive and rarely done.

When cells don't get what they need, regardless of what's in your blood, they don't operate or replicate properly. They also send out an alarm signal to the body that they are starving. This constant starving signal creates low-grade anxiety in the system. It also causes the cells of our body to start preparing for imminent danger. The cells begin to store whatever they have, toxins included. It doesn't discriminate as it figures that *something* is better than *nothing*. The body grows in dysfunction and toxicity, further compounding the struggle and expediting the dom-ino effect. The body will even build fat cells, for as long as it can, just to store the toxins it thinks it might need if worse comes to worse.

Trace mineral resources

Currently, the two best trace mineral supplements I have found are "Superior Fulvic Humic Concentrated X935" and "Mother Earth Labs Humic & Fulvic SC." These two brands commonly come up in the personal reading work I do. The Superior brand seems to be slightly better but seems to be poorly impacted by fluoride. Since almost every municipality in the United States fluoridates its water, this poses a problem. This issue is also evident if you use fluoride toothpaste or mouthwash. If you are on well water or can verify that your water filtration system removes fluoride, and you don't use fluoride products, Superior is the one I would take. It's a liquid, dosed by drops into water, and allows you to reduce the dosage if needed. It is never recom-mended that anyone exceed the suggested dosage. More is not better when it comes to trace minerals. Consistency matters more. If you can't be certain, your water is fluoride-free, then the Mother Earth Labs SC is suggested. It comes as a pill or as a liquid added to water and seems less affected by the fluoride content. The liquid would still allow for lower dosages if needed.

Keep in mind that as the cells become properly supplied with trace minerals, it is very likely that they will uptake more of any supplementa-tion you're already taking. They can also increase the uptake of medication. Make sure you're paying close attention to your own system, know the symptoms of overdosing on your meds, and work with your doctor to ensure the choices you're making are right for you and your well-being. The good news about greater uptake and functionality, though, is that this often means you can reduce what you're taking or eventually completely remove it from your protocol. If you suspect you may be toxic, try starting at a low dose and gradually working to a full dose. This can help prevent a quick toxic dump from the cells as they start absorbing what they need.

Cell salts and hydration

The "twelve essential cell salts," as they are commonly termed, are the other piece of the foundational puzzle that allows us to maximize our potential. There are 26 or 27 total cell salts, depending upon which research you're looking at. Of those, twelve are considered crucial to proper cellular function. Most importantly, among those benefits is the cell's ability to pick up and utilize water! The effects of dehydration at the cellular level are catastrophic and widespread and wreak just as much havoc as a trace mineral deficiency.

The body uses water in so many critical ways. It is how we eliminate toxins from the system, how we lubricate tissues, and as part of the cell-to-cell communication capacities of the body, just to name a few. If your cells are dehydrated, they can't clean themselves, function as they should, or replicate in healthy ways. Most people believe that drinking more water is the solution to dehydration. While more water in the system is sometimes called for, the more common issue is that our body simply cannot absorb that water into the cells themselves due to a deficiency in these twelve cell salts. If a person is deficient, the fluids they drink simply run right through their system, excreted as urine, having never actually had the intended influence on hydration! Sometimes the unabsorbed water will be found in between the cells instead, causing the inflammation so many people struggle with. Odd as it may sound, one of the solutions for water-retention inflammation is to hydrate properly by addressing the cell-salt issue. Like a trace mineral deficiency, dehydrated cells cannot absorb properly. Most people are dehydrated, even those who drink a lot of water!

Addressing this is simply a matter of taking a supplement. Though many options are available when searching for cell salts, they do not always contain all twelve. It is my experience that these lower-count varieties are not as effective. Unlike trace minerals, the quality of cell salts seems to be more standardized. This allows each person to choose the brand and options that they like best. Personally, I use Hyland's

Bioplasma. It's good quality, effective and inexpensive. It also allows me to titrate my dosage more easily since it suggests taking it thrice daily. Rarely do I see someone who needs that much, me included, so I can still use it when my need decreases by simply taking one or two instead.

Your potential, in every aspect of your Being, is affected at a foundational level by core trace mineralization and the ability to be properly hydrated. When brought back into balance, these two simple things make monumental changes in the entire system. They also create a proper foundation for all other work you may do towards reaching your own potential!

Key takeaways to implement

* Take trace minerals like by the brand "Superior Fulvic Humic Concentrated X935" or "Mother Earth Labs Humic & Fulvic SC"

* Take 12 essential cell salts: Bioplasma by the brand "Hyland's"

In general, I recommend following the bottle's dosage, *more is not better,* and more could even create problems.

I have found that some children can benefit from taking trace minerals. You can schedule a reading with me to ascertain your child's needs or contact the manufacturer for dosage for children.

About the author

Julie North is an internationally renowned Medium and Medical Intuitive who offers her unique services to seekers of positive transformation during these intense times of evolutionary change. Gifted from birth with the ability to communicate with Guides as well as hear/see energies and other sentient dimensions, she is a sought-after spiritual advisor, teacher and speaker.

Julie's heart is aligned in the tradition of native medicine, integrating work with all living things, physical and non-physical, honoring the alignment between humanity and Mother Earth for *The Greatest Good of All That Is*. She has a long history of mentoring and teaching both teens and adults who are awakening their intuitive, psychic, and empathic abilities and wish to deepen their skills. She assists them in learning practices that create personal balance and effect positive change in both their Inner and Outer Worlds.

Julie has been the keynote speaker at events such as "Council Grove Conference," CAM events for doctors and those in medical professional fields, the *A.R.E. Midwest Annual Conference*, and multiple international retreats and spiritual events. She also facilitates in-depth workshops, intensives and meditations from her home base in Central Ohio as well as around the country. From 2013-2018, Julie was the Ceremonial Center Director for "Rootwire," a transformational music and arts festival, where she led opening/closing ceremonies, as well as curating a broad spectrum of educational opportunities covering personal development, meditation, spirituality, movement/martial arts, leadership, sustainability and other growth-oriented topics.

Through all these areas of focus, Julie's goal continues to be the ongoing empowerment of each individual through clarity of purpose, truth of intention and the honoring of all things.

www.julienorth.com

Part Three

Inner Tools

Seth brings heartfelt passion and grounded purpose to everything he does, offering compassionate, practical tools to help others navigate life's most challenging transitions. Rooted in the belief that moving from survival to true fulfillment is not only possible but powerful, his methods empower people to heal, lead, and live with intention.

In addition to his transformational work with adults, Seth also writes award-winning children's books that foster empathy, resilience, and emotional awareness from an early age.

— Book momma Chandra

6

Frameworks for Facing Hard Times

Seth Eliot

wareness is the path. Resilience is the journey. Together, they
unlock the bridge to your highest potential.

In my work as The Psychic Bridge, I guide people through
the most profound journeys of their lives: the journey to release their
hidden truths, confront the unseen forces holding them back, and step
boldly into the authentic version of themselves. Whether it's through
connecting with spirit, navigating unresolved grief, or untangling emotional and energetic wounds, I help people move beyond pain and
confusion to clarity, purpose, and resilience.

Think of awareness as the bridge — a glowing pathway inviting you
to cross into a deeper understanding of yourself and your potential. Resilience is the process of crossing that bridge: facing the fears,
uncertainties, and challenges along the way while discovering the truth
that you've had the strength within you all along. Together, these two
forces create the foundation for transformation, not just in your own life
but in the lives of everyone you touch.

In this chapter, I'll dive into how awareness and resilience work together to create the foundation for human potential. I'll introduce you to
three powerful frameworks I use with my clients — individuals who are
ready to uncover the truths they've been carrying, heal from the wounds

they've endured, and step into the next chapter of their lives with confidence and purpose.

The Six Levels of Awareness: These levels: metacognition, inner awareness, self-awareness, social awareness, organizational awareness, and world awareness — offer a comprehensive framework for understanding yourself and your interactions with others. By cultivating these layers of awareness, you enhance your emotional intelligence, adaptability, and sense of purpose, driving both personal and professional growth.

The SMILE Method: This method takes you on a journey through current day emotional healing, from the shock of an experience to partial acceptance, navigating overwhelming emotions, and engaging in deep learning. It moves you from mere resistance to fully embracing and evolving from your experiences, enabling profound personal growth.

The GRACE Method: This method provides a transformative approach to healing past wounds and challenging experiences. Through deep introspection, taking responsibility, processing emotions, and cultivating compassion, it empowers you to move beyond understanding and forgiveness to active, enthusiastic growth, and lasting transformation.

These tools aren't just theoretical concepts — they are grounded in my work with countless clients who have faced the fires of grief, trauma, and uncertainty and come out the other side stronger, clearer, and more aligned with their true purpose. As The Psychic Bridge, my role is to help you navigate this journey with intuition, insight, and unwavering support, so that you too can discover what's possible when awareness meets resilience.

This chapter isn't just about theory; it's about action. It's about giving you the tools to not only see the bridge but to cross it — to step into the version of yourself that's waiting on the other side. The journey won't always be easy, but I promise it will be worth it. As you grow and transform, you'll naturally inspire and uplift those around you, creating a ripple effect of positive change that extends far beyond yourself.

Are you ready to take that first step? Let's embark on this journey together and discover what's possible when awareness meets resilience. The potential is limitless. Let's dive in!

Awareness

What is awareness?

Awareness is the gateway to transformation. It's the ability to truly know yourself — your emotions, triggers, values, and behaviors — and understand how they shape your interactions with the world. By cultivating awareness, you gain clarity about your internal states and external environment, allowing you to grow, connect, and make empowered decisions.

Why is awareness important?

Awareness is the foundation of human potential. It provides the insight needed to overcome challenges, build resilience, and align with your purpose. By seeing where you are, where you've been, and where you're going, awareness becomes the catalyst for personal growth and meaningful change. It's what allows you and I to evolve as individuals, professionals, and leaders.

Awareness is all about restoring your freedom to choose what you want instead of what your past imposes on you.
— Deepak Chopra

The Six Levels of Awareness

The Six Levels of Awareness — metacognition, inner awareness, self-awareness, social awareness, organizational awareness, and world awareness —create a framework for growth and transformation. Each level deepens your understanding of yourself and your place in the world, fostering emotional resilience, authentic connections, and purposeful action. Together, they empower you to thrive in all areas of life.

1. Metacognition

Metacognition is the awareness of your own awareness. It's about knowing what you know, recognizing what you don't, and understanding how to navigate uncertainty. By being conscious of your strengths and weaknesses, particularly in learning and leadership, metacognition allows you to refine your skills and continuously improve.

2. Inner awareness

Inner awareness is understanding your internal world — your emotions, reactions, and baseline contentment. Ask yourself:

- Am I in touch with my feelings?

- How do I process adversity?

- What is my default state of joy, play, and optimism?

Exploring these questions enhances your insight into your inner self, guiding personal growth and balance.

3. Self-awareness

Self-awareness is about how you show up in the world — at work, home, and in relationships. It's a reflection of your strengths, weaknesses, and how others perceive you. Ask trusted friends or colleagues to describe you. If their responses align, it shows consistency in how you present yourself and highlights areas for celebration or improvement.

4. Social awareness

Social awareness focuses on understanding the relationships that shape your life — self, family, romantic, and professional. Reflect on how these connections have evolved and how past experiences influence your current dynamics. By exploring these relationships, you can foster growth and transformation across all aspects of your life. Shifting how you engage with others begins here, and that shift is powerful:

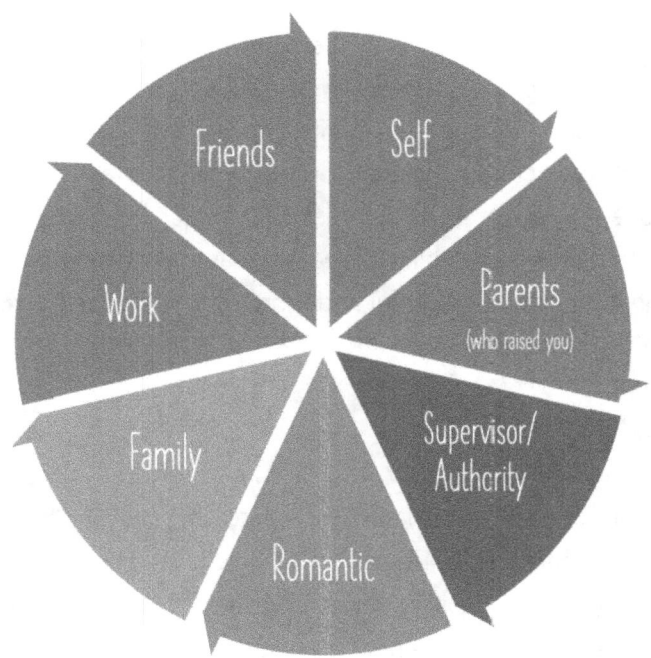

5. Organizational awareness

Organizational awareness is about looking beyond yourself to understand group dynamics, whether in teams, workplaces, or communities. It involves emotional intelligence — reading a room, anticipating needs, and meeting people where they are. By recognizing that each person is a unique work of art, you can build stronger, more empathetic connections and collaborations.

6. World awareness

World awareness is the understanding of global challenges and the human experience at large. It's about embodying love, kindness, and compassion amidst the world's hardships. By striving to be the change you wish to see and paying it forward, you contribute to a ripple effect of positive transformation.

Choice is everything! Awareness provides you and I with the freedom to choose. A choice for how to choose wisely! A choice for how to RESPOND instead of REACT. The next time adversity walks into your path, pause, take a deep breath, pause again, and respond accordingly. Use your awareness and respond in a different way. Every day, every choice is new opportunity to change the rest of your life and the easier it will be to objectively review, analyze, and make a better choice moving forward. For any situation, you can take a breath, reframe your thoughts, and re-invent the future with thoughtful and more insightful choices.

Resilience

What is Resilience?

Resilience is the ability to face and overcome challenges, adapt to change, and maintain well-being in the face of adversity. It's about bouncing back from setbacks, learning from difficulties, and emerging stronger. Resilience isn't just enduring hardship — it's thriving through it, drawing on inner strength, emotional intelligence, and support systems to navigate life's uncertainties. Like a muscle, resilience grows stronger the more it is used, preparing both you and I to respond to future challenges with greater ease and efficiency.

Why is Resilience important?

Resilience is essential for unlocking human potential. It empowers you and I to adapt, stay motivated, and transform challenges into opportunities for growth. By regulating emotions and managing stress, resilience fosters clear decision-making and emotional well-being. It strengthens relationships, builds empathy, and encourages personal and professional growth. Ultimately, resilience fuels confidence, enabling you to take risks, innovate, and pursue meaningful goals, unlocking your full potential in every aspect of life.

The greatest glory in living lies not in never falling,
but in rising every time we fall.

— *Nelson Mandela*

The SMILE Method

The SMILE Method helps people gain awareness and a deep understanding of their individual healing process, which occurs *directly following* trauma or unexpected news of any type. This healing method helps people move through challenging times in the present moment.

1. Shock

This is unavoidable. This is nature's first line of defense to protect the mind, body, and soul from the event occurring in the present. How cool is it to think that, as humans, our bodies are equipped to prevent you and I from living in startling and emotionally charged chaos for too long? How cool is it to think your body has the capacity to regulate the amount of information being processed at any one single time?

2. Mock-cceptance

Part denial. Part acceptance. It is the pause between the painful event *and* the pain itself. It is where one day you might feel on top of the world and, the next, you might not be able to get out of bed. You do what we need to do, finish what you need to finish during this phase, perhaps not even remembering how exactly you accomplish this. Your body, mind, and soul here start allowing the information to start trickling into your psyche one day at a time.

3. In Overwhelmdom

These are the significant and poignant emotions that you and I must venture through to get to the other side. Here, you encounter frustration, anger, sadness, loneliness, despair, feelings of lack, and more. Allowing yourself to fully experience these emotions is crucial for releasing your attachment to the event itself. During this phase, your body, mind, and soul are given the space to process, release, and ultimately, let things be as they are.

4. Learning

This is where you reflect, sitting with everything that has happened. It will be tough, raw, and messy. Yet, with this awareness, you learn to do better next time. This phase is crucial because it helps you release the tight grip we all hold on emotionally charged events. Here, the body, mind, and soul work together to shed the excess weight and heaviness of the experience, creating space to breathe freely once more — perhaps even deeply.

5. Embrace

After all the hard work of the previous phases, this is where you get to exhale and surrender. It's like coming home at the end of a long journey. Here, you fully accept what has happened with grace, strength, and dignity. You may even find yourself feeling grateful for the opportunities and new perspectives that this emotionally charged event has brought into your life — possibilities that might not have existed before. Some might even call this ... freedom.

This five-step method is the key to your survival. I might even say it is the key to your success and thriving in this crazy modern world. This process is not easy. It is no picnic. It is not always linear. It is not going to be sunshine and rainbows. It will be messy. It will make you cringe at times. You will want to give up. Don't! Stay with it. Don't just "trust the process," nope! I want you to be the process. Own the process. Make it your little *bitch!*

This entire process is filled with ups and downs. You will get through this! It will be the best of times and the worst of times. It will set you up for success time and time again in the future. It will provide endless opportunities and possibilities — ever when you are convinced the world is ending around you. It will be laced with signs from the universe you are where you are supposed to be. It will help you on your journey to your highest self, your self-love, and your greatest potential as a human.

If you stay the course and move through each phase, you will be *way* more confident in who you are. All change in this world starts with you. All shifts in this space begin with your first thought, then feeling, and then action.

Consider this: When you know better, you do better. When you know what's coming, it makes the whole process easier to manage your way through it, or at least move through the process.

Sometimes your joy is the source of your smile, but sometimes your smile can be the source of your joy.
— *Thich Nhat Hanh*

The GRACE Method

If the SMILE Method is for awareness and navigation through adversity and trauma in the present moment or not-so-distant past, then the GRACE Method is for breaking free from the past, letting go of your conditioning, and moving beyond. All this, so you can reframe your past, embrace your present, and create a better future and legacy for you and everyone around you. The GRACE Method helps you move beyond your past, move beyond pain, and start moving onward.

This method provides a structured approach to deep healing, emotional release, personal accountability, and growth, offering a comprehensive path to overcoming past challenges and evolving into a more authentic and resilient self.

1. Going deep

For every event that happens, there are three sides to the story (yours, the others', and what really happened). Am I right? In this phase, you must explore, be vulnerable, and let your guards down with a selected few that you love and trust. You get to exaggerate the hell of your side of the story to them. Afterwards, though, you get to reach inside to a place of vulnerability, honesty, and empathy as you share the others' side of the story. Here, you stretch yourself, remove your ego, and leave your own judgments, thoughts, and prejudices in order to stay objective, truthful, and present. This is a very powerful process. Stay with it.

2. Responsibility

Once you understand the truth, as best you can, without prejudice, you are then ready to discuss responsibility. This is where you take accountability for your participation in the event. Here is where the bitter truth comes out whether you are prepared or not. This is where preparation and transparency meet. This is where you uncover your part in all of this and how you contributed. This is tough. Be honest. Be culpable. Be open.

3. Activate (your emotions)

Remember those significant and poignant emotions in the In Over-whelmdom stage in the SMILE Method, well here they are again. This is where you activate all your emotions. You give yourself permission to release all that you have been holding inside, all that you have left unsaid, and all that you never said. Let the emotions flow. Acknowledge those feelings. Here is your not-so-subtle reminder that life is messy, and emotions can be chaos. Be gentle. Be gracious and be patient with yourself. You deserve it.

4. Compassion

After the beautiful and unprecedented series of storms called emotions, here is where the hardest work of all begins. Compassion is acceptance. Compassion is forgiveness. Compassion is understanding. Compassion is one of the most challenging and rewarding gifts to receive, to master, and to give unto others. Similarly, forgiveness can truly move mountains of traumas, angers, and hatred within seconds. It is fierce and powerful. In this phase, compassion will help you forgive even the most egregious of offenses and/or offenders in your life, including yourself.

5. Evolve

At the end of the day, we are all works in progress. You and I are here to remember our light, grow, reflect, expand, and develop into who we are without pretense of ego. It is here where you find the confidence, courage, and strength to move onward, in life, with passion, enthusiasm, and zest. It is important because if you don't evolve, you don't progress. If you don't learn from your mistakes, then you are doomed to repeat them. If you continue doing what you've always done, you will continue to get what you've always gotten, right?

Adulting is hard. This five-step method is the key to longevity as a human species. As stated above, I might even say it is the key to our human success and thriving on Earth. Similarly to the SMILE Method, this work and these exercises done here are not for the faint of heart. It takes bravery, incredulous inner strength, and the desire to be the best version of yourself you can be. Luckily, however, this process will not only serve you results immediately, but it takes much less time than the SMILE Method.

If you and I as people do not evolve, then the laws would never change, minds would never shift, and then life would be stagnant, boring, and inconsequential.

Now, go and break free from your past, so you can start living a refreshed life. And, go and rewrite your past, so you can embrace a new you.

It doesn't matter who you are, where you come from.
The ability to triumph begins with you. Always.
— *Oprah Winfrey*

A little story

This year has been one of the toughest of my life. The Big D: divorce. From the moment I made the decision to end my marriage, through the grueling legal process, it has been a journey of pain, heartache, and profound emotion. Living under the same roof for four long months after that initial discussion only amplified the difficulty (and trust me, I've learned that's too long for me). But it wasn't until the day I moved out that the full weight of it all hit me. I felt lost — numb, sad, and deeply entrenched in what I now know was situational depression.

Then, amidst my emotional roller coaster, the universe intervened. I was invited to speak at two conferences in Los Angeles — one on the SMILE Method and the other on the Six Levels of Awareness. I couldn't have known it at the time, but those talks would become my lifeline, pulling me out of my darkest moments (I called it a funk) and guiding me back to the light.

For thirty days leading up to the conferences — both talks serendipitously scheduled for the same day — I immersed myself in the work. Each day, I reviewed the talks in detail, repeating the messages of awareness, resilience, and healing. Little by little, those daily reminders became more than preparation — they became my practice. Moving through the daily adventure, of applying the Six Levels of Awareness, provided me the fortitude and bravery to face each day with courage and seek support, joy, and laughter. The constant reminder was something I didn't even know that I needed. Similarly, knowing that divorce is one of the most stressful and challenging experiences, taking myself through the SMILE Method daily became my anchor and provided me the hope and confidence to persevere and to process my emotions and travel the path from survival to thriving!

I didn't realize it at the time, but those talks were the gift I desperately needed. They reminded me of the power within me — the power to heal, to persevere, and to rebuild. Now, I offer them to you. These tools helped me navigate my toughest storm, and I hope they can do the same for you.

Opportunities & possibilities

Imagine a world where every person has faced their inner battles, shattered their limitations, and emerged stronger, more aware, and resilient. A world where you and I choose our responses with intention and love, creating a ripple effect of positive energy that transforms everything it touches. A world where collaboration fuels innovation, empathy drives connection, and resilience turns every challenge into an opportunity for growth.

You and I have all walked through shadows of pain, loneliness, and shame, carrying burdens that felt insurmountable. But those shadows are not the end of your story — they are the fuel for your greatest light. When you rebuild your foundation with awareness, resilience, and grace, you don't just survive — you thrive.

We are the ones we've been waiting for.
We are the change that we seek.
— *Barack Obama*

Now is your time. Wake up each day and hunt for joy like it's the most precious treasure. Find grace in the smallest moments and live gratitude as a way of life. With the tools and wisdom of the SMILE Method, GRACE Method, and the Six Levels of Awareness, you are equipped to face any storm, conquer any challenge, and embrace every opportunity for growth.

Every moment is a choice. Will you choose to see possibilities in adversity? Will you transform setbacks into setups for comebacks? Will you be the light in a heavy world? If you do, you won't just change your life — you'll inspire those around you to do the same.

Imagine a world where every person awakens to their true potential. A world where healing is contagious, hope is our common language, and together we elevate the human experience to extraordinary heights. This isn't a fantasy — it's a choice you and I can make, starting now.

The best is yet to come, and it begins with you and I. Together, let's build that future — boldly, with hope in our hearts and hands ready to create.

It is not the strongest of the species that survive,
nor the most intelligent, but the one most responsive to change.
— Charles Darwin

Remember this:

1. Elevating awareness is your path, and strengthening resilience is your journey.

2. Grief doesn't change you — it reveals you. Do the work and embrace the rewards of breathing deeply.

3. Break free from your past and reframe your present to pursue joy, play, and hope. Reimagine your future to build a legacy worth leaving.

As you stand on the edge of transformation, remember: You hold the keys to your evolution. Awareness is your compass, guiding you to deeper self-understanding and authentic connections. Resilience is your strength, empowering you to rise above challenges, heal wounds, and grow from every experience. Together, they are a powerful duo capable of reshaping your life and inspiring others.

By integrating the Six Levels of Awareness and the SMILE and GRACE Methods into your life, you take charge of your story, rewriting it with intention, compassion, and courage. Change begins within — when you choose to see every challenge as an opportunity, every setback as a lesson, and every day as a chance to grow.

The path may not always be easy, but it will always be yours to choose. Choose wisely. Choose courageously. Choose to be the light, the change, and the inspiration the world needs. Every moment is an opportunity to create a ripple of positive change.

Let's co-create a world where awareness and resilience lead both of us to our highest selves and most extraordinary futures. The journey begins within you and I. Are you ready to begin?

All this work is a movement toward the greatest human potential possible.

Will you help me spread the word?

Key takeaways to implement

At this point, you have been saturated with loads of information. You're probably like, "Seth, that's all great information, but what am I supposed to do with that? What's the next logical step for me?" Here are three logical next steps for you to take immediate action in your lives.

* To elevate your self-awareness, try this powerful exercise: write an email or make a good old-fashioned phone call to twenty to thirty people in your life — those you trust, respect, and value. Ask them to share their honest feedback on your strengths, weaknesses, and unique gifts, both personally and professionally. These could be co-workers, bosses, friends, or family members. Let them know this is an opportunity for you to gain deeper insight into how you show up in the world and to grow from their perspectives. Embrace their feedback with an open mind and heart; it's a step toward becoming the best version of yourself.

* If there's something in your life that you haven't fully processed yet, take a moment to pause and reflect. Identify where you are in the journey and review the SMILE Method to see which phase resonates most with your current experience. Acknowledge this stage and recognize your progress — no matter how small. Celebrate how far you've come and express gratitude for the growth you've achieved. Remember, there's no set timeline or "right" way to move through these phases. Give yourself grace and trust that you are doing your best. Everyone moves at their own pace, and that's perfectly okay.

* Is there something in your past that you just can't get past? I challenge you to share your story — your side and the other side! Find a trusted confidant, someone you love, respect, and who is free of judgment. Ask them to help you work through a difficult experience that still weighs on you. In a comfortable space, tell them your side of the story — exaggerate, be dramatic, and express it fully. Then, take a deep breath, perhaps make some tea, and return to share the story again, this time from the other person's perspective. Be honest, transparent, and honor their experience — even if the "other side" is someone who has passed or a previous work situation.

* After sharing, take a moment to breathe, close your eyes, and reflect. Then, ask your confidant what they noticed about the second version. Discuss their observations and your feelings about the process. By the end, you'll gain a deeper understanding of what happened and be ready to continue your work with Responsibility in the GRACE Method.

About the author

Seth Eliot Santoro, CEC, is a globally recognized Speaker, Smileologist, Psychic Medium, and Spiritual Consultant dedicated to helping people fulfill their creative, professional, and personal potential by releasing the hidden truths holding them back. Known as The Psychic Bridge, Seth guides individuals through personal, emotional, and spiritual transformations, empowering them to heal old wounds, align with their purpose, and thrive with resilience and clarity.

Seth provides a space for self-discovery and empowerment through his Release Your Truth philosophy. By combining profound spiritual insight with practical strategies, he helps clients navigate challenges and embrace bold authenticity by confronting hidden traumas with an unmatched depth of insight into their spiritual selves. Seth's compassionate guidance speaks to those on the cusp of transformation—whether they're overcoming relational struggles, career transitions, or unresolved family dynamics. His work, especially impactful within the LGBTQIA+ community, is rooted in believing that everyone can reclaim their truth and confidently create the life they desire.

As a five-time international bestselling author, intuitive leader, and sought-after speaker, Seth inspires audiences worldwide to connect with their inner power and pursue their dreams fearlessly. His unique ability to sense the unseen and merge spiritual understanding with real-world wisdom positions him as a thought leader in personal growth. With Seth, releasing your truth becomes the key to unlocking resilience, clarity, and a life of greater joy and purpose.

iamsetheliot.com

Diana's energy, presence, intuitive knowing, and confidence are immediately striking. Her education on Human Design has proven in my own life to be invaluable for understanding our unique energetic blueprints and decision-making processes.

Her chapter reflects the depth and care she brings to her work.

— *Book momma Chandra*

7

Discovering Your Human Design: Where It All Begins

Diana Elizabeth

We come into this world carrying a seed — a living code that holds our unique genetic imprint. Within it lives our specific gifts, strengths, ancestral material, and the key lessons we're here to integrate as part of our evolution. This chapter is where your remembering begins.

Human design: A portal to your truth

The primary tool I use is Human Design — a cutting-edge, practical, transformational, and empirical system that brings together science and ancient tools. It's a synthesis of quantum physics, neutrinos (subatomic particles that emanate mainly from the sun, traverse the planets, and imprint us with information), the Chinese I Ching, the Kabbalah Tree of Life, the chakra system, and cosmology.

Human Design is a portal that leads you directly to your differentiated self, your uniqueness — so you can stop chasing who you think you should be and start living as who you are.

Another powerful gift of Human Design is its precision. While therapy can take years to uncover the root of your struggles, Human Design targets them directly. Many of my clients come to me after years in therapy — still spinning, still searching. Human Design goes straight to the heart of what is yours and what's not, revealing your blind spots, patterns, and core vulnerabilities. That's why I often say it's like an X-ray of yourself.

It offers more than just awareness. It gives you a path to realignment a way to reclaim what's yours, release what isn't, and work with both your strengths and sensitivities with clarity. This isn't a system of belief — it's a lived experiment one that leads you back to the truth of who you are.

A jewel for children

Human Design is a tool that serves everyone, regardless of age. That said, I find it especially invaluable for children. Why? Because children are fresh energy. Instead of molding them into who the parent thinks they should be, parents can begin to nurture and empower their child's uniqueness from the very start.

This process begins with the parent. The more you understand your own design, the better equipped you are to support your child's journey — free from projection, control, or unconscious interference.

When parents have this knowledge, it becomes an invaluable resource, helping them honor and celebrate their child for who they truly are, rather than imposing external expectations. It fosters presence, permission, and a deep trust in the child's natural unfolding.

The vehicle you were born with

Let me make this clear: we are all spiritual beings — expressions of the same Source. While we share a common origin, we come into life with distinct energetic blueprints, each carrying a unique pattern of lessons and potential meant to guide our growth and evolution.

Now, imagine that each of us is born with a specific kind of vehicle — designed to move through life in a particular way. If you're a Ferrari trying to go off-road just because others are doing it, you'll end up feeling stuck, frustrated, or even broken. But when you understand how your vehicle is designed — how it's meant to move — you stop forcing. You start flowing.

Where it all begins: Your type

This is where the journey begins: with your Type. Your Type is your vehicle. Your energetic architecture. And understanding it is the first key to living in alignment.

In this chapter, I'm going to cover three fundamental pieces to get you started in discovering and empowering your uniqueness:

- **Bioenergetic Type** — How you're naturally designed to operate.

- **Aura** — How your energy speaks before you do.

- **Strategy** — How to engage with life and others in ways that honor your nature. (It works in tandem with your Inner Authority, which guides decision-making, though we won't dive into that here.)

These are not just starting points — they're the foundation. When embodied, they unlock the momentum that comes from honoring your true design — less resistance, more flow.

As you go deeper into your design, key elements like your Inner Authority, Profile, Centers, Channels, and Gates offer richer insight into how your energy is meant to function. Each layer is significant. You can preview these in the example image on the next page — but it all begins here: with your Type.

Bioenergetic Type: Your natural way of operating and honoring your being and energy.

Aura: Your presence. It speaks before you say a word.

Strategy: How to be "in relationship with" life and others in ways that honor you. Works in tandem with your decision-making authority.

Inner Authority: How to make decisions that are truly yours.

Profile: Your role in which you actualize yourself as your type.

Defined/Colored Centers: What you emit out to the world, what is consistent in you, your strengths.

YOUR HUMAN

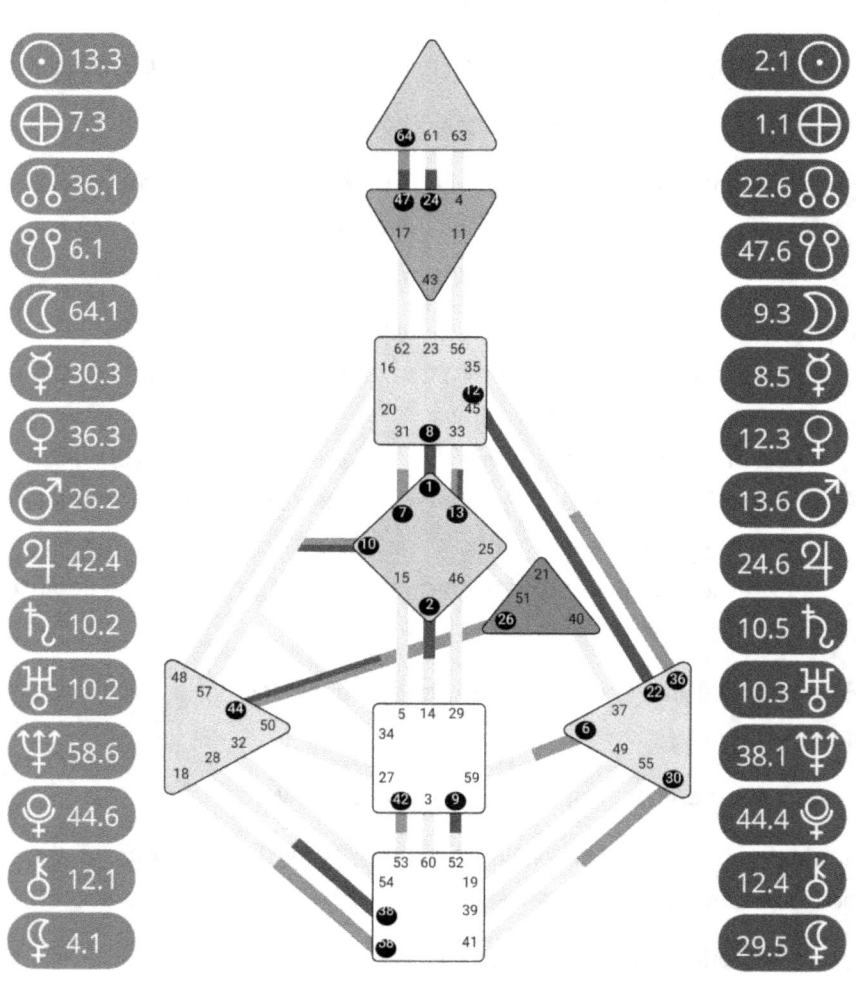

DESIGN CHART

Type:	Manifestor
Signature:	Peace
Not-Self:	Anger
Strategy:	To Inform
Authority:	Emotional
Profile:	1 / 3
Definition:	Triple Split Definition

Incarnation cross:
Right Angle Cross of The Sphinx (2/1 | 13/7)

Undefined/White Centers: The conditioning you take in from the environment and others. What is inconsistent in you, your vulnerabilities yet your greatest sources of wisdom.

Planetary activations - Gates and Channels: Specifies your uniqueness, gifts, strengths, key lessons, and purpose **(Incarnation Cross)**.

Nodes of the Moon: Mathematical points. Marks where you have been which is what you will be redefining and working on in your first 40 years of life as your base. And where you are going, which marks the 2ⁿᵈ stage of your life.

The design and personality side: The design side is everything that is in red, it is **unconscious** in you, and it is working at a body level, it is what you bring from your ancestry, your tree. The personality side is everything that is in black, is conscious in you, it is what you can recognize in yourself.

Definition: Connections of your defined/colored centers, your energy flow.

Note: Each part holds specific meaning, and together they reveal the full picture of your unique design.

Extracting your design

In Human Design, there are **five Types** and **four Auras**, each with its respective Strategy.

The Types are:

1. **Generator**, with its subtype

2. **Manifesting generator**

3. **Projector**

4. **Manifestor**

5. **Reflector**

To extract your HD BodyGraph, visit https://e3-portal.com/human-chart/.

Under the Human Design tab, input your name, date of birth, and include your **exact** time and **place** of birth. This calculation is time-sensitive, so refer to your birth certificate for accuracy.

Once you've identified your Type — and that of your kids, partner, family, and friends — head to the relevant section below to explore what it all means and begin the process of remembering who you truly are.

Generator and manifesting generator (MG)

As a generator or MG, you are designed to be a master builder and creator. You have natural sustainable energy to build and achieve mastery of the work and crafts that you absolutely love. Generators constitute 36 percent of the population and MGs 34 percent of the population. Together, you are the energetic engine of the world. You quite literally keep it moving.

Your Aura is impersonal, enveloping, and magnetic, it naturally attracts life to itself.

Strategy: To respond

Your strategy is to respond via a guttural yes or no, body expansion or contraction to what your magnetic aura is naturally attracting.

What is your magnetic aura attracting into your life becomes your key question.

In order for your aura to attract nourishing opportunities for your gut to respond to, it is key for you to create a fertile field of response around you. You do this by raising your vibration. Your vibration sets the frequency from which your Aura is attracting life to you.

As a generator and MG, you are responding to an external reality, not an internal reality. This means that you must experience it through one of your five senses in your outer reality for your gut to respond. This is not your mind responding, it is your gut and your body that responds to external stimuli. If it lights you up at a gut/body level, it's for you, if it doesn't, it's a no. Can you honor the wisdom of your gut/body? Your gut is your one and only guru. Your gut is your guide, it leads you to what is correct for you. There is no mind involved in this process.

Your magnetic aura is doing all the work for you; it is attracting life to you. All you need to do is respond. To respond, you must be in the now to register your gut response. Can you surrender to your now? This is where the reprogramming awaits you.

For decision making, ensure you respect your strategy and inner authority.

Difference between generators and manifesting generators:

Because MGs have manifesting capacity, they are more energetic, they are like a tornado at level 10, while the generators are also like a tornado but at level 5.

- MGs are dynamic, they are natural multitaskers, and it is correct for them to skip steps as it is part of their efficiency; they also have the capacity to adapt to the next task quickly and easily.

- *Generator's* rhythm is progressive, one step at a time, and they go through natural periods of plateaus.

Key advice for generators:

After you start on X (project, work, or study) that your gut/body has responded with a hell yes — you will find yourself plateauing. Know this is normal, ensure you embrace your plateaus, and don't abandon your craft. This is a key time where integration takes place, which will move you to the next level. This is how you become a master creator and builder of your craft. If you abandon it, you won't become a master of anything. Be resilient in your plateaus.

Key advice for manifesting generators:

Because of your natural dynamism, it is imperative that you don't start (things, activities, projects) out of pure impulsivity, take a little time to register in your gut/body your yes or no response prior to involving yourself in activities. Otherwise, you will find yourself running around like a chicken without a head, involved in so many activities and pursuits from pure impulsiveness rather than an aligned response. In the end, this impulsive action will lead you to degeneration on all levels. Respect your precious well of energy.

Note: The level of impulsivity will vary depending on each person's unique mechanical configuration in their design.

Work and health:

You have the natural, sustainable energy to work a 9-to-5 — and more.

The key is to give your energy only to the work, projects, or activities your body has said *yes* to — in other words, to what lights you up at a gut/body level.

If you are not doing the work you love, you will degenerate yourself. You will get to 50 years old feeling frustrated, exhausted, out of energy — burnt out and disconnected. Generators and MGs make up 70 percent of the population, this is why most of the world lives in perpetual frustration because they are giving their precious energy to jobs they don't love.

Go to bed only when you are tired, in other words, when you have exhausted all your energy. If you have energy left and you force yourself to go to sleep, you will have a hard time falling asleep, you will wake up throughout the night and get low-quality rest.

Don't waste your precious energy compensating for your vulnerabilities.

Instead, use your Human Design to understand them — so you can extract wisdom from those places, rather than letting them pull you out of alignment.

To honor the generators and MGs in your life (including children):

Ask them yes or no questions, this gives them the opportunity to respond with their gut. Their gut response is their truth.

Give them options. Do you want to go to the movies with me? Do you want to go to the park with me? This is key for you to put in practice with your generator and MG children so they can begin to build a relationship with their body and register their gut response.

Respect their yes or no response and don't ask them why they said yes or no. There is no mind or rationalization involved in their yes or no response. Remember, it is their gut response, not their mind response.

You can stimulate them to play and get involved in activities that are correct for them by asking them yes/no questions.

Don't impose demands on them, ask them yes/no questions, and give them options instead.

Parents of manifesting generator children:

If you are the parent of a MG child, and, for example, they try soccer for two weeks and they don't like it, it is correct for them to abandon, don't force them to finish the program. Remember how their energy works: if they don't love it, they will degenerate themselves. They are designed to easily adapt, to quickly move to another task, they are highly dynamic. As a society we have been conditioned to finish the activity we started, this conditioning will deteriorate your MG child as it goes against their essence.

Because MG children tend to be very energetic, parents will often think they have ADHD and will start medicating them, when the reality is that their hyperactivity is part of their inherent nature.

Instead, teach them to connect and register their body response via the art of asking them yes/no questions and by giving them options. From this space they can begin to filter activities that are correct for them.

There are other aspects of the BodyGraph that can also predispose individuals to hyperactivity which can be misread as ADHD.

Generators and MGs: When you are in flow with your energy, you experience satisfaction. When you are not, you experience frustration. Frustration is your signal for realignment.

Projectors

Projectors, you are the new models of the world, you make up 20 percent of the population. You are designed to be natural guides to others, as well as mediators and coordinators of group success.

Your Aura is laser-focused, penetrating, and absorbing. At an aura level, you penetrate right into the core of the other and absorb them right into your being. This gives you the natural capacity to guide them as you have direct insight into who they are, their gifts, and their limitations.

Strategy: Recognition and invitation

As a projector, you are naturally geared to guide and help others because of your natural ability to see right into them. But the dilemma is that if you have not been properly recognized and invited to give your guidance, advice, and gifts, then you will waste your precious energy talking to a brick wall. Here is where bitterness stems for you.

As a projector, you must first recognize and value yourself, and all the precious energy and attention that you naturally put into the other, you need to redirect it to yourself first.

Being a projector is all about *presence.* When you recognize, love, and value yourself along with your gifts — then this is what you will project out; naturally attracting the recognition and invitation of those who are correct for you.

What to do as you wait for the recognition and invitation:

Given that your strategy is to wait to be recognized and invited to give your valuable guidance and gifts. The best thing to do in the time of "waiting" is to focus your energy on working on yourself, doing what you love, discovering and sharpening your natural talents and gifts, and putting them on display once they are polished, all while trusting that those who are meant for you will recognize you.

You are not here to chase. You are here to be chased.

The dilemma with the projector is that they have great insight into who the other is, but not into who they are.

This is why it is imperative to invest in getting to know yourself and your gifts because the recognition and invitations you receive must be of who you are, and not of who you are not. This is how you differentiate who sees you for you — or who just wants your attention. HD helps you directly see what is *you*, in other words, what is consistent in you.

For decisions on which invitations to take on, follow your inner authority.

Health and work:

As a projector you do not have sustainable generating energy. It is imperative to have ample rest throughout your day and time alone to cleanse from the energy and impressions you have picked up and amplified via your undefined and open centers.

You are designed for work and activities of short duration and focused concentration.

You're not here for long hours of sustained physical work — your energy isn't built for that. You're here to be compensated for the deep guidance and insight that only you can offer.

Learn to recognize in your body when enough is enough and when to stop. You naturally amplify the energy of generators which can have you working like a slave and lead you to burn out, if not aware.

Don't feel guilty for taking time to rest; it is part of honoring yourself. Solitude is your medicine to come back to your center and reorient. Go to bed prior to being tired or exhausted.

To honor the projectors in your life (including children):

If they seem pushy, wanting to give you unsolicited advice or guidance, don't take it personally, their intention is to help you.

Recognize them and invite them. Your recognition must be authentic.

Ask them for their insight or opinion. You have a natural guide by your side.

Encourage and respect their alone time to rest, cleanse, and reorient.

Parents of projector children:

Your projector child is more sensitive and dependent. They need more TLC and personalized attention. Recognize their goodness. Honor their time to rest. Teach them about recognition and invitation. Projector children who receive the recognition of their parents are healthy adults.

Projectors: When aligned with your being, you experience success, and when not aligned you experience bitterness. Bitterness is simply your signal for realignment.

Manifestor type

Manifestors constitute eight percent of the population. Yet this is the type that most parents push their kids to be, going against the essence of 92 percent of the children in our world.

As a manifestor you are designed to be a trailblazer, a proactive and independent leader. You are designed to initiate, innovate, transgress limitations and standardized models, as well as impact, catalyze, and mobilize others into their greatness.

As a manifestor you need *freedom!* Freedom to initiate from your deep inner urges in all aspects of your life. To filter what initiations are correct for you, you must follow your inner authority.

Your aura:

Your aura impacts, protects, and is impenetrable; at an aura level you are pushing the other out of your way.

Your aura naturally does this so it can clear the path for you to do what you came here to do: *initiate* and *create!*

When you are rooted in your authentic power, others who don't know you are a manifestor will sense the impact of your powerful aura and will personalize it; they will either withdraw or be magnetized toward you.

Your impactful aura, by its very nature, awakens the vulnerabilities and insecurities of others; and/or your aura highly moves and inspires them. This happens without you saying a word. The more you are in your power, the greater the effect.

An unaware manifestor will internalize the withdrawn response of the other and think that there is something wrong with themself; leading them to either people-please, isolate, or provoke — when it is just their aura doing its thing. Your aura naturally moves the other out of your way, it protects you and is impenetrable because you are not here to be influenced by others. All you need to do is keep being yourself, those who are for you will respect your impact and will be open to your catalyzing initiations — and those who aren't, won't, and that's okay. Remember your aura naturally awakens the vulnerabilities in others.

As a manifestor, you impact with what you have defined in your chart, in other words with what is consistent/inherent in you.

Strategy: To inform

Because of your powerful aura, your strategy is to inform. Prior to acting on a decision that has been filtered through your inner authority, you need to inform only those who are going to be directly affected by your decision. Informing does not mean asking for permission. It is simply a strategy to prepare others who will be affected by your initiation and action to help minimize resistance. You are only informing as courtesy, not asking for permission.

Work:

It does not suit you to work where you are not leading or where you don't have the freedom to initiate and create.

You have tremendous starting power to initiate new catalyzing action, new projects, and new creations that emanate from your inner urges (not your mind). But you don't have the generating energy to sustain your initiations in a consistent way.

This is why it is important to give yourself ample rest, learn to delegate, if necessary, and have the correct allies, which are chosen via your strategy and inner authority and consist of mutual respect for each other's nature.

After you have given your potent energy to initiating and creating, you need to retreat and rest, until the next inner urge moves you to initiate and create again.

In a metaphoric sense, you are made for sprints, not for marathons.

It takes courage to step into your inherent manifestor power, and for you, the concept of rejection needs to be redefined.

Health:

It is key to get ample rest in your daily life as you do not have sustainable or generating energy. You require a lot of downtime not only to recover but also to cleanse from the energy you have picked up and amplified from the generator type.

Go to bed prior to being tired or exhausted.

Learn to recognize in your body when enough is enough and when to stop. You naturally amplify the energy of generators around you, which can have you working like a slave and lead you to burn out, if not aware.

Because you don't have natural sustainable energy, don't over-demand this from yourself and compensate with gallons of coffee or energy pills. Respect your natural energy flow!

To honor the manifestors in your life (including children):

The biggest gift you can give them is Freedom. The freer they feel, the best of themselves they will give!

Respect their independence and privacy. Allow them the opportunity to initiate. Inform them. Keep them in the loop on anything that involves them. A relationship with a manifestor is about presence.

If you have an empowered manifestor in your life, they are teaching you to be secure in yourself.

Children:

Manifestor children pose a natural insecurity to parents and teachers because of their transgressing and independent nature. This is the reason why many adult manifestors in today's world have jailed their power and are either submissive, provokers, or have isolated themselves because since childhood they have been controlled or restricted.

As a parent, you can begin to honor your manifestor child by understanding that they don't need to be stimulated to play or act. They stimulate themselves in their own activities.

Give them the freedom to initiate, move, and create. Respect their independence and autonomy. Don't control them.

Teach them courtesy and to ask for permission, this will serve them later with their strategy to inform.

If you say no to their request, ensure you are sensible in explaining your reasoning.

Manifestors: When aligned with your being, you experience peace, and when not aligned, you experience anger. Anger is simply your signal for realignment.

Reflector type

Reflectors are a minority, making up only 2 percent of the population. Reflectors, you are designed to be one with our totality. Your greatest potential by design is to evaluate the energetic well-being of others, groups, the environment, and society. You are designed to share your objective perspectives and wisdom to help others and society recalibrate into a more balanced, harmonious, and healthier state.

Reflectors have no definition; you are completely open.

Your aura:

Your aura is much like a scanner, it scans and samples the energy of the environment and of others. Because of this capacity, you are designed to be a natural detector of the health and fluctuations in the environment, as well as of what and who stands out from the multitude with their authentic differences.

Because of your openness, your nature is always changing, much like the cycle of the moon. You honor your essence when you accept and embrace your ever-changing nature, and perspectives, and delight in the surprises you naturally detect and witness in others and in the environment.

The key for a reflector is to not identify nor attach to what their aura is naturally scanning and sampling. Otherwise, you can live a very overwhelming, emotionally chaotic, and confusing life. Embracing your openness in a detached way and giving yourself ample time to process is what allows you to understand diversity. This approach is what enables you to help recalibrate others and society with your impartial and objective perspective.

Strategy:

Given you have no definition, your strategy and decision-making authority come via a totally different process which is tied to the moon's cycle.

Reflectors are very sensitive to neutrino impact, and it takes them a moon cycle, approximately 29 days, to gain clarity on decisions that are correct for them.

Learning about your own activations in your BodyGraph and the timing of the moon is crucial for you.

To honor the reflectors in your life (including children):

If you have a reflector in your life, include them, and ask them to share their views, but don't expect them to agree with you. Why? Because reflectors who are in alignment with their being will give you an impartial and objective perspective.

Children:

Give them access to the world so they can begin to sample diversity. Don't pressure them to make decisions, give them time. They see the world in a more neutral and detached way. They need lots of alone time. Time in nature is extremely balancing for them. Teach them that there are no good or bad things, but rather different things.

Reflectors: When aligned, you experience the beauty of surprise, and when not aligned, you experience disappointment. Disappointment is only your signal for realignment

---

Now that you've been introduced to the essence of each Type, it can be helpful to step back and see how they work together — how each one plays a distinct and essential role in the bigger picture.

Think of it like the process of creating a movie.

The **manifestor** is the producer — the one who gets the vision off the ground, initiating momentum and bringing something new into the world.

The **generators** and **manifesting generators** are the actors, the film crew, and the editors — those consistently doing, building, and refining the vision into reality.

The **projector** is the director — guiding the process, recognizing the talents of others, and aligning everything.

The **reflector** is the audience — the mirror. They show how well the movie landed and offer deep insight into the impact of the whole.

Each role is essential. When you truly understand your Type, you stop trying to fit into roles that were never yours to begin with. You stop pouring energy into what drains you — and start aligning with what's naturally yours to give. That's when your true impact begins to unfold.

The Invitation

I teach Human Design to empower you. To help you align with your unique direction — not through rigid systems, but through deep awareness.

When you truly understand your design, you don't just gain insight — you gain tools. Tools to:

- Work with your vulnerabilities

- Optimize your strengths

- Release what's not yours

- Love and accept yourself — radically, deeply, and completely.

In relationships, this understanding changes everything. You stop taking things personally. You start seeing others through a new lens — one of compassion, respect, and empowerment.

So, I invite you into this process of self-recognition.
To honor the seed within you.
To free it from distortion.
And to let it flourish, just as it was designed to.

It has been an honor to share this foundational piece of Human Design with you.

And remember there is more!

Key takeaways to implement

* Go to https://e3-portal.com/human-chart/ to generate your Human Design chart.

* Identify your Type and Strategy.

* Read the respective section in this chapter that applies to you.

* Contact me for more information and guidance.

* Begin experimenting. Begin observing.

* Start honoring your uniqueness — and that of your children, too.

About the author

Diana Elizabeth was born and raised in the Sierras of Northern Peru, where the mountains, mystery, and simplicity of life first awakened her sensitivity to what lies beneath the surface. From a young age, she sensed that life carried deeper truths —ones that couldn't be explained by logic alone, but could be felt, known, and remembered.

Though she followed a traditional path and earned a degree in Business Management, her deeper calling never left her. It moved quietly beneath every choice, pulling her toward what was real.

When Diana discovered Human Design in 2015, it wasn't just a system — it was a remembering. It gave form to what she had always known and named truths she had long lived. It didn't show her something new — it confirmed what had always lived within her, with a precision that felt like coming home. And soon after, she began guiding others to do the same.

She went on to complete four years of professional training to become a certified Human Design Analyst, followed by advanced specialization in Life Cycles and Relationships. Her work blends intuitive depth, practical insight, and lived experience — meeting each person where they are, and pointing them back to who they've always been.

Today, Diana guides individuals, couples, families, and business leaders to understand the unique design they were born with — not just for insight, but for transformation. Her work is an invitation to return to inner authority, to raise empowered children, and to build aligned teams that thrive beyond conventional models.

To her, Human Design is a living, breathing compass that roots you in your truth and power, so you can live aligned and unapologetically as the person you were born to be.

e3-portal.com

Teresa genuinely embodies the unconditional love she teaches, channeling this energy through her presence and practice in ways that transform those around her. Her meditation approach is accessible to anyone seeking to connect with love's transformative power in their daily life.

Teresa demonstrates that love isn't just an emotion but a force that can reshape our experience of ourselves and our world.

— *Book momma Chandra*

8

Live in the Frequency of Love

Teresa Rodriguez

Love alone is capable of uniting living beings in such a way as to complete and fulfill them, for it alone takes them and joins them by what is deepest in themselves.
— *Pierre Teilhard de Chardin*

To be in love is the most incredible feeling in the world. When you're in love, everything in your life feels incredible. Everything feels enhanced. You have more energy. You feel euphoric. You're driven to succeed. You forgive easily. You feel so wonderful and amazing because love is the most powerful energy that exists.

Everything is energy. You are energy. Your thoughts are energy. Your feelings are energy. And so is love. Energy fields intertwine with each other. Everything is connected. This is basic physics. Even though you may not see energy, you can feel it. You can't see gravity. You feel it. You experience it all day, every day. It isn't solid. You don't touch it. Yet it exists.

Your body is made of energy. It consists of about seven billion atoms. An atom is made of protons, neutrons, and electrons; energy. We are spiritual beings having a human experience. Your spirit, your soul, your very essence is made of energy.

Your thoughts, feelings, and actions create an energetic ripple. What you think, how you feel, and what you do affects the health of your body and the health of your mind. It's such a great time to be alive. The next wave of the human potential movement is here. And you are part of it, my friend.

Your mind and your thoughts are extremely powerful. I learned to limit my news decades ago because of a wellness program. I worked in the administration of a fire department during the attacks of September 11, 2001. Just after that happened, we were put through a wellness program. We were told to limit our news because our brains don't know the difference between watching something on TV and experiencing something in real life. Our brain and body react to what we watch on TV as if we are living that experience. That means you will have more anxiety, feel more stress, and experience more depression, especially if you repeatedly watch negative things like the news.

If you watch the same negative stories over again, you get the adverse effects over again. And if you practice using the energy of love over again, you will get the beneficial effects over again.

That's why I focus on cultivating the energy of love from the moment I wake up. That's why I suggest you do this too. Love uplifts, heals, and inspires. Love serves as the greatest empowering force that exists. Sometimes, love can feel like a complex emotional experience, but it doesn't have to feel that way. You are happy beyond measure when you're aligned with love. You can use the power of love to enhance your life and really get the best out of your human experience. I'm not talking about romantic love. Although romantic love is pretty damn awesome. I highly recommend you learn to navigate that type of love, too. I'm talking about applying the frequency of unconditional love to all areas of your life.

I say God for the ease of describing; infinite source, divine, universe, energy of unconditional love, or whatever name you use as our highest source. I use the name of God because it is easier than listing out all the options. Please insert what resonates with you.

God knows we aren't perfect. I'll be the first to tell you I'm not perfect. Sometimes I say the wrong things. Sometimes I do the wrong things. I don't always realize what I've done until someone else points it out. Sometimes, I learn a hard lesson, and it feels like a big slap in the face. Hard lessons are part of our experience so we can grow into the person we truly want to become. But because I put into practice what I'm about to guide you through, my heart is always in a place of love. I always intend to help people and never intend to hurt them. I sincerely acknowledge and apologize if I've done something that hurts someone. I do my best to make right what I've done. Then, I do my best to move forward with love.

Those kinds of hard lessons happen when I let my ego get in the way. When you're aligned with love, and you put your ego aside, that's when the magic happens. That's when you recover from challenges fast. That's when you feel energized and motivated. That's when you do things that you think are impossible.

I come from a pretty traumatic background. I'm not the only one. I venture to say that you've experienced trauma, too. I used to keep everything to myself. I opened up to close family members and friends in my late teens. Then, as I got older, I opened up to friends who weren't as close. Then, I opened up to clients I coached and women I mentored. After so many years of sharing my experiences, I realized how important it is for me to share.

When I was a teenager, I struggled with self-worth, depression, and drugs. When I was really young, I thought it was normal to have the police come to my house because my dad got drunk and hit my mom. The first time I tried pot, I was five. When I was about six, I went to school in slippers with my hair in a bird's nest of a crazy mess. My 12-year-old sister was left in charge of my older brother and me. It was one of the times my parents were separated. I remember the teacher looking at me with an expression I didn't understand. She looked like she felt so sorry for me. I felt fine. It didn't seem like anything was wrong or out of the ordinary. But she insisted on calling home.

My dad lived somewhere else at the time, and I'm sure he was at work anyway. My mom was with her boyfriend. We were left on our own a lot when things were rough. Even though it felt wrong, I didn't know anything else. We did what we had to do to survive. I'm not going to go into too many details about my childhood. I'm open and upfront about my life. You can find me on multiple podcasts sharing details. I have a number of written works in different places, too. But in this chapter, I'm going to talk with you about a meditation I've pieced together from 20 years of experience and a simple breathing technique that I use to help myself navigate old pattern that sometimes wants to resurface. I practice these two things every day so I can live my best life through hard times. I also practice them so I can feel as if I'm floating on air during the good times.

One of my mentors told me something to help me stay aligned with God when I'm having a conflict with someone. He wanted to give me a scenario so I would think about the pain the other person is going through, and I can make my decisions based on the big picture. He told me what I'm about to tell you so I can stay true to myself and who I am no matter what. I think about what he said almost every day. I'll give you the scenario now.

Imagine you are sitting on a chair outside of a pool with your back to the water. And someone keeps splashing you. Imagine you don't want to get wet. You can't see them even if you turn your head because there's furniture in the way. You continue to get upset and your anger is building up. Now imagine getting really mad and getting up from your chair. You move toward the pool to tell them to stop. Once you can see them, you realize that they are drowning. The whole time you were getting upset, they were splashing because they were out of control and drowning. That changed your perspective, didn't it? It changed your reaction. You immediately changed from being angry with them into taking action to help them.

Now imagine if, instead of being angry when you were splashed, you stayed curious. Instead of reacting with a knee jerk, you wondered what was happening and moved toward them with curiosity. Imagine keeping that energy for yourself that was wasted by being mad at another person. That's what focusing on love will do for you. You'll stay curious. You'll spend less energy on anger, fear, bitterness, and resentment. And more energy on fun, joy, fulfillment, and adventure.

The meditation I guide is based on the intention of unconditional love, which I believe is the energy of God. The energy of love has the power to help you in ways you may not have thought. It will help you regain peace and thrive during your most challenging times. I use the breathing technique multiple times throughout my day, and I use the fundamentals from the meditation as a way of life.

Once you learn how to use the fundamentals of this meditation in your everyday life, you will learn to notice the patterns that get in your way. You'll learn to let go of petty things and feel really good most of the time. I say most of the time because you're here to grow and experience all aspects and feelings of life. It's just what you're here to do. Cultivating love from the moment you wake up will help you notice negative patterns when they show up.

We are conditioned from birth. Our conditioning has been repeated generation after generation. Only some of us learn to break that conditioning. And those conditions try to creep up, especially when you're faced with a serious challenge.

I still project my feelings onto the people closest to me. It's something I own. It's something I face every day. Don't get me wrong, my hard work has paid off. I'm completely different than I was 20 years ago. Now when I'm projecting my feelings, I watch it happen as if I'm watching from the outside. I struggle the most when I'm tired or stressed. It's just the way it is. It's a pattern I continue to break. You'll need to break patterns that get in your way. If you want to truly live, it'll be important to learn to be vulnerable, communicate effectively, and give unconditional love. Those three things are what I work on now and what I will work on every day for the rest of my life.

I've also learned that the longer you work at changing your behavior pattern, the easier it becomes to have better behavior. You build character. And when you have strong character, you bounce out of old patterns faster and smoother as time goes on. The best thing to do is to stay consistent. If you veer off, gently bring yourself back and give yourself grace. You get to be you, imperfections and all. There's beauty inside of you. You're unique. You have gifts to offer the world. There's a reason you're reading this right now. The reason is because you know there's more to life than working to live. You know in your heart that you want more out of life than resentment, anger, and bitterness. You truly want to be happy, fulfilled and loved. And you get to be your unique self, spread your gifts, and do you. That's why you're alive.

I wasn't sure I wanted to have kids until I was about 30 years old. Parenting is one of the toughest jobs around. The best job but one of the toughest. When I finally decided to have kids, I did everything I could to break my dysfunctional pattern. I promised myself if I ever had kids, I would put every ounce of energy I had into being the best parent I possibly could.

I took parenting classes, saw a child psychologist, and read a ton of books on parenting. I watched every parenting skills video I could find. I surrounded myself with other parents doing the same things. I practiced and practiced having patience, being kind but firm, and keeping our communication open so we could always work together no matter what.

And I still make mistakes. I still lose patience. Sometimes, I have to remind myself that I had kids on purpose. I know if I had the chance to do my life over again, I would make the same decision about having kids in a heartbeat. Being the best parent that I possibly can has led me to do what I do. It's led me to find the power of unconditional love. It's led me to you. I know who I am because of my kids. I love my life and everything that happens to me because of them. It's been a tough journey and it's been so wonderful too. I'm grateful for every moment.

Most of us have been brought up with conditional love. Most people only know how to love under conditions. It's entirely different to love someone unconditionally. When you give love to someone without expecting anything back, that's real love. That's unconditional love. Now remember, love says "no," and love has boundaries. Loving someone unconditionally doesn't mean giving up your rights as a person. It doesn't mean giving up your emotional health. It doesn't mean you let someone hurt you physically. You learn to have healthy boundaries out of love for yourself and others. You learn to be yourself. You learn to love yourself. Because when you live in alignment with love, the people who aren't the right kind of people will disappear from your life. They drop off somehow. Maybe it's you that leaves. You'll repel the people who don't belong in your life when you live your truth. And that's a good thing. That's what you want.

When I think back to the tough times I've had, I look back with gratitude. I'm grateful, and I feel so much love for everything that has happened to me. Because when you put yourself in the energy of love, you feel better. You inspire. You are inspired. Everything feels possible. You're healthier and happier. You're willing to live life to the fullest. Think about how happy and healthy you feel when you truly feel loved. It's easier to move through the ups and downs of life when you're aligned with love.

I implemented giving the intention of love first in meditation and then into my everyday life. I learned about the benefits of intention from experiments done by Lynn McTaggart. In her book, "The Power of 8" she proves how small groups of people can heal others with their thoughts and, in turn, heal themselves. She explains that when you heal others, you, in turn, get better. You don't just get better. You heal on a bigger level than the people you are intending to heal. She points out that the moment you stop thinking about yourself, the miraculous power you have to heal your own life gets unleashed. It's a beautiful cycle. And it works.

Meditation is important. But the real work is done when you take the fundamentals of meditation to your everyday life. And it is a million times worth the effort. Intentionally giving unconditional love will give you energy, passion, and drive to break down barriers. Once you learn to continually give love, you'll stop yourself from putting certain barriers up in the first place. You'll learn to get out of your own way.

Unconditional love meditation exercise

The way this meditation, this way of life, works is by you sending the energy of unconditional love to someone else. I'd like you to take a few minutes and give a simple version of it a try right now. It's easy. All you have to do is think of someone you'd like to send unconditional love. They don't have to know you're sending it to them for this to work. They can be anywhere in the world. They can have passed away. You can think of two people that are in conflict with each other. If you want to get really deep, think of someone you're having a conflict with right now. It could be someone from your past, and you're no longer in touch with them.

Start to pull energy from the top of your head and take it down to your heart. Bring this energy in from Source straight through your crown chakra to your heart chakra. This loving energy you will give won't just come from you. It'll come from God. You aren't alone in your journey. You have an Infinite Source guiding you, loving you, and supporting you. So, pull the energy in from the Divine and get into the feeling of love as much as possible. Really feel it. Feel as if you're receiving the most incredible hug from someone with all of their being, and you're giving them the exact kind of hug back with all of your being. It feels so overwhelmingly wonderful to get and give a hug like that. I don't know if you've ever had a hug like that, but there's nothing like it.

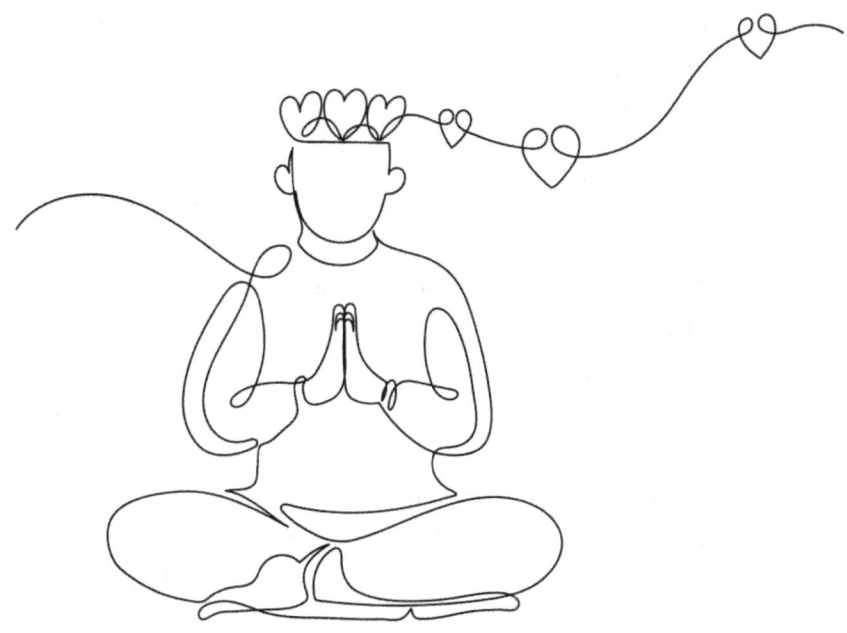

The most important part of this exercise is to feel love as deeply in your mind and body as possible. Love is the most powerful energy that exists. After a few moments of building up the energy of love in your heart, send it energetically to that person. Send it knowing you may not get thanked. Send it without expecting anything back. Genuinely give love for the sake of giving it because you want to help. Sending unconditional love will make a difference in that person's life. It will make an even bigger difference in yours. I recommend doing this for 20 minutes every morning.

Once you use this practice in meditation and in your everyday life, you're going to feel a huge shift. You're going to start to see through the eyes of love. You're going to be open to receiving more love. You're going to be happier and healthier. You'll have a better relationship with yourself and others. It'll be easier for you to laugh and enjoy your life as much as possible.

There are those moments when you may feel bad. Those moments when it's hard to feel happy. I mean, that's what being human is all about. We're here to experience and grow. And for the times that are the toughest, I recommend putting breathwork into practice. Without breathwork, I'd be an emotional mess. Practicing breathwork keeps me from giving a knee-jerk reaction and gives me the sense to respond with a balanced mind. Again, I'm not perfect. Don't expect yourself to be either. This is a practice. It's a wonderful practice. The more you do it, the easier it gets. And if you don't get it right, acknowledge that, apologize if necessary, and move on with love.

I learned the basic counting of this breathing technique from Theresa Bullard. She is a physicist, author, and speaker. Theresa bridges the gap between science and spirituality in easy ways to understand and apply. The basic technique is from her, and I've added my own touch.

Breathing technique exercise

Now that you know the basic method for meditation, let's have you try the breathing technique. Before you start, let me say while you breathe in, imagine the energy of love coming in from the top of your head from Infinite Source. When you hold your breath imagine that energy stopping at your heart. And when you let your breath out, circle the energy back to the top of your head.

OK, now here's what you do: Breathe in for five seconds. Hold your breath for five seconds. Exhale for 10 seconds. Again, when you breathe in for a count of five, breathe in the energy of love. When you hold your breath for the count of five, hold the energy of love in your heart. And when you breathe out for 10, give the energy love. Now circle back with your breath to the top of your head and bring more love in from the Divine. You're going to do this breathing technique for a round of five. Once you do a round of five of these breaths, your mind will be calmer. Your body will feel more relaxed. Do it as many times as it takes to get centered again. Feel free to do it throughout the day.

Imagine being able to bounce back from an intense conversation quickly. Imagine reaching the outcome you want. Imagine being able to navigate challenges without feeling anger or resentment. The more you practice this, the easier it becomes to resolve conflict with yourself and with others. Now, this isn't a magic pill. You won't get instant results. You will get results over time and with consistent practice. Those feelings of anger, bitterness, and resentment may surface. That's OK. You'll learn to let them go. You can't feel angry or resentful if you're feeling love. It's just not possible. When you live this way, you will do the most amazing things. You won't let petty or deep-rooted issues get in your way. You will feel the magic of love in every way possible. You will be happy, and you will enjoy your life the way you're meant to enjoy it.

Key takeaways to implement

✳ Unconditional love meditation exercise

Think of someone you'd like to send unconditional love.

Start to pull energy from the top of your head and take it down to your heart. Bring this energy in from the Divine Source straight through your crown chakra to your heart chakra. Pull the energy in from the Divine and get into the feeling of love as much as possible. Really feel it. Feel as if you're receiving the most incredible hug from someone with all of their being, and you're giving them the exact kind of hug back with all of your being.

The most important part of this exercise is to feel love as deeply in your mind and body as possible. Love is the most powerful energy that exists. After a few moments of building up the energy of love in your heart, send it energetically to that person. Send it knowing you may not get thanked. Send it without expecting anything back. Genuinely give love for the sake of giving it because you want to help. Sending unconditional love will make a difference in that person's life. It will make an even bigger difference in yours.

I recommend doing this for 20 minutes every morning.

✳ Breathing technique exercise

Breathe in for five seconds. Hold your breath for five seconds. Exhale for 10 seconds. Again, when you breathe in for a count of five, breathe in the energy of love. When you hold your breath for the count of five, hold the energy of love in your heart. And when you breathe out for 10, give the energy love. Now circle back with your breath to the top of your head and bring more love in from the Divine.

You're going to do this breathing technique for a round of five. Once you do a round of five of these breaths, your mind will be calmer. Your body will feel more relaxed. Do it as many times as it takes to get centered again. Feel free to do it throughout the day.

About the author

Teresa Rodriguez is an Intuitive Life Coach. She is the founder and CEO of 8th Dimension Pillars, LLC. When you work with Teresa you learn to trust yourself. You learn to develop and continue to enhance your intuition. You learn to align your life with the energy of unconditional love. Work with Teresa to become the person you are meant to become. For more information of how to work with Teresa, visit:

8thdimensionpillars.com

Mac embodies nature's raw power in his being, Elemental Embodiment lives within him. From Pacific Ocean cold plunging to primal workouts, he moves as a conscious force of the elements. Mac continues his family legacy of the Human Potential Movement nurtured at Esalen while honoring the native peoples' connection to that sacred land.

The nature-based practices Mac shares in his chapter are foundational to well-being.

— *Book momma Chandra*

9

Right Relation through Elemental Embodiment

Mac Murphy

When I am connected with nature, I feel grounded by the earth, cleansed and invigorated by the water, clear-minded with an expanded breath from the air, and my passion and joy ignited by the fire; I have the ability to flow and rise above the challenges of life. This informs my thoughts, my movements, and how I interact with others. This practice invokes power, grace, and compassion for all life.

We human beings are not separate from nature, though we have built a material divide that disconnects us from our source. In this time of technological advance and the neglect of the natural world, I believe it is of utmost importance to remember and practice the old ways of our ancestors in how to live in right relation with nature: right relation meaning to honor and respect Mother Nature. We once lived in harmony with the Earth as a species and it is in our human potential to return to that right relation.

Often, I feel overwhelmed by the churn of society. I feel like an alien in cities that have snuffed out the vibrancy of nature. When I am disconnected from the natural world, I experience anxiety, depression, and fatigue. With all the impacts of technology that the human body takes on, much sickness derives. The air is polluted by fossil fuels and there are man-made toxins that rain down on the Earth.

I imagine you may be similarly aware and perhaps you are asking, "What can I do?" My answer: Use the practices I share below to practice and bring Elemental Embodiment into your life.

The source of all life

I channel my strength and energy from nature. It's a practice of consciously connecting to the source of all life. In this unique alchemy that these four elements create together, life is possible. Many of us have forgotten that we are made of these key ingredients. To invoke the key ingredients is at the core of Elemental Embodiment.

Without connection to source comes existential terror

I am concerned for the Earth and all life, as the environmental crisis continues. Earth is in the sixth mass extinction and our timeline is limited for a potential sustainable future. Those of you thinking of this, like me, are likely feeling existential terror like I am.

What I see is that species are dying off and archaic habitats are being destroyed.

I cannot help but ask: Why are we killing our source of life? What are we leaving for future generations? How many mental, physical, and emotional symptoms and diseases are a product of not living in accordance with the cycles of nature?

Remedies to avoid extinction of Earth and life:

- Cultivate a personal and intimate connection with nature to bring you into right relation, aligning your choices as an individual and inspiring others to do the same.

- Answer the significant need for change in how we humans interact with the Earth. Shifting to renewable energy resources, regenerative farming practices, stopping overfishing, and deforesting the planet.

- Honor the widespread need for ecopsychology which is the inter-disciplinary field that focuses on the synthesis of ecology and psychology and the promotion of sustainability.

Call to ecopsychology

Ecopsychology focuses on studying the emotional bond between humans and the Earth; for the health of the greater ecosystem of the Earth that has no borders. It acknowledges how collective human health is affected by the increasing impact on the planet; there is a call to action, a cry for embodied activism.

Beyond volunteering with environmental organizations and beach cleanup efforts, you and I need to cultivate a deeper connection with the power of nature and all life. We must cultivate curiosity and mindful practice in relation to the natural world.

Prayer and spirit as the doorway

We have the opportunity to learn from our native people all over the world. If you look, as I have, you would see how they lived in right relation to the natural world, in a relationship of honor and respect. A commonality in all earth-based cultures is prayer.

There is spirit in the land. The Earth's land has consciousness.

There are many ways we can give back to the Earth.

Prayer and expressions of gratitude are core to reciprocity with the land. I encourage you to speak to the land about what you are grateful for. This means creating a physical and energetic dialogue with the elements.

I invite you to begin to relate to them as Grandmother Earth and Grandfather Sky. We are a product of Grandmother and Grandfather. Each human is the living embodiment of all who came before. Our bodies are made of the earth, air, water, fire, and the granules of stars beyond. To invoke our ancestors is to pay homage to the will of the divine which is embodied in the land and in the flesh of all living things, aligning with right relationship.

My practice of Elemental Embodiment
invitation to you

My practice of what I call Elemental Embodiment is a lifestyle and a daily practice. It connects me, and you, to all life on Earth and the cosmological forces that influence the spin of this planet that we are a product of. Attuning to the cycle of the moon and to the change of seasons are core to this practice.

There is an invitation from nature to align ourselves and our activities with these cycles. When you and I accept the invitation through attuning to the seasons and moon cycle, the body, mind, and spirit cultivate well-being, much like a healthy ecosystem.

Understanding how the processes of the body work in relation to cycles of nature is a valuable concept to grasp, when your mind begins to grasp it then your energy and actions follow. You can ground, which means consciously connecting to Earth's gravity, and begin to pull up the life force into your body. Everything is energy, where the mind goes energy flows. Take in the elements, interact with them, and channel them through you. Once you cultivate the discipline to engage them, they are free. The following pages describe the core practices of Elemental Embodiment.

Lineages of ancient medicine practices and divination such as Traditional Chinese Medicine, Ayurveda, Taoism, Astrology, and Shamanism are designed to bring harmony to the body in relation to the elements and the spirit world. They are rooted in observing nature in relationship to self and the collective.

I spent seven months at the Five Immortals temple studying Taoist practices in Wudangshan China, under the direction of Li Shifu of the Pure Yang and Dragon Gate Sects. We had a rigorous schedule in the temple – wake up an hour before sunrise and then run to the top of Bai Ma Shan, White Horse Mountain. There at the Shen Wu temple at the mountain's summit, I practiced Yang Sheng Gong, Longevity Qi Gong with the rising sun. Facing the east, we practiced these ancient movements with the rising yang qi of the sun. There were mountain peaks all around and waterfalls poured down their faces; it felt like being in ancient China on the mountaintop, invigorating and connective.

These millennia-old embodiment practices balance and harmonize the energy (qi) of the body. They connect the vessel of the human body with the earth below and the heavens above, much like a tree is rooted in the ground and reaching up toward the sun. From this rooted place, we can breathe and move the structures of the body, filled with life-giving breath, and intentionally send energy through the meridians, nourishing our organs.

Many systems of Qi Gong have been channeled by the great masters to create balance in our relationship with the elements.

In Chinese Medicine, there are five elements, wood, fire, earth, metal, and water. Some movements may be for balancing one's fire, for example increasing heat in deficient bodies, and decreasing heat in excessive bodies. There is much to investigate in these ancient alchemical and primordial practices, to utilize the power of the medicine of nature.

Our human ancestors have evolved through much elemental hardship. Through ice ages, drought, famine, competition, and predation from megafauna over human history we have cultivated a resilience in combating and surviving through what modern people see as harsh conditions. We humans have these genetics in us to persevere and even thrive through the challenges that the natural world presents. With the comforts of housing, heating, and automation many of us have lost touch with the resilience that our hunter-gatherer ancestors relied on for survival, we have become soft and often suffer because of this.

How do we reignite those genetic pathways to cultivate healing and resilience in our body vessels? We must challenge ourselves. What doesn't kill us makes us stronger. *"Hormesis."* Hormesis I define as the adaptive process in the body of producing beneficial chemicals and hormones after the exposure to elemental stressors.

Since a child, growing up on the Pacific Ocean, I developed a fondness for the cold of the ocean. I started my conditioning early. I remember as a child I could swim in the ocean for long periods, playing in the waves. The cold invigorates, activating the nervous system.

Embodied Biomimicry

Biomimicry means to observe nature and mimic it in our design of technology and materials — much like applying the wings of birds to airplanes, the resiliency of caves to stone houses, and the waterproof fur of otters to wetsuits. Embodied Biomimicry is achieved by observing nature and animals in action, we can apply their traits to our own inquiry into embodiment. For example, I observe a swell in the ocean, billowing along in its current, it builds into a wave, crests, and a wall of water is exposed and with a mighty force, it crashes creating a froth of chaos, then stills on the shore.

I can apply this to my movement. An undulation in my spine, creating soft mobility in my body, and then building to a lengthening, a reaching, and then a jumping; landing into a squat, transitioning into rest on the ground. Observe animals in motion, how they stalk or swim, and mimic it in your own way. This practice hones our ability to be like nature. Like Bruce Lee says, "Water can flow, or it can crash. Be water, my friend ..."

I call this Embodied Biomimicry in the practice of Elemental Embodiment. The elements offer so much to us in their raw forms and as metaphors to learn from. Embodying them is part of this great remembering, rekindling our connection to the source of nature.

Elemental Embodiment of wood, fire, metal, water, and earth

Each element offers many teachings and practices to enhance our human potential. I will now express what each element offers the seeker if we choose to deepen our intimacy with them. This is inspired by the Five

Elemental Theory from Traditional Chinese Medicine and my own investigations of Native American traditions. Elemental Embodiment is a lens to relate to the natural world and to our bodies' well-being and potential. It offers insight into who we are prone to be in body, mind, and spirit, in physical form and personality. Below is just a taste of this theory and practice.

To deepen one's connection with nature and receive the medicinal therapeutic effect, it is essential to take the time to sit still in the presence and take in the beauty. Notice the colors of the surroundings, see the different shades of earth tones and greens. Be in awe of this miracle of life that you are an extension of. Smell the scents in the fresh air. Feel the earth below supporting you. After sitting still for long enough in silence, notice the birds that return. Listen to their song. Notice how it makes you feel. See how the light peers through the trees and where the shadows are cast. Take in the vitality of nature through your senses and be nourished by it.

Wood

Starting with the wood element there is an invitation to relate to all of plant life. Wood is the energy of rooting down into the earth, pulling up the minerals and waters below, growing them, and expressing through branches and flowers to the sky. Wood governs the eyes, tendons, liver, and gallbladder. It represents the direction of the east, the color green, the rising sun, the season of spring, birth, and the emotion of anger.

To balance wood:

- Stand amongst trees and look into the vastness of greens is a balancing practice of the wood Element.

- Face the east and reflect upon your birth and what wants to be born within yourself.

- Scream and produce sounds to release the stagnation of anger from your liver.

- Have plants in your home or have a garden.

- Tend to the birth of seeds, nurture the roots of plants, and thus nurture yourself.

- Face the east and pray to what is being born and send gratitude to the spirit of nature for your birth.

Forest medicine

In Japan, there is a practice called Shinrin-Yoku, or Forest Bathing. It is a therapeutic experience where one spends time in nature and meditates on the senses taking in the natural environment.

Forest bathing exercises:

- Interact with the plants in riparian zones. Look deeply into their verdancy aka their greenness.

- Smell spring flowers and wild herbs; learn their names and medicinal properties.

- Look at the roots of trees in how they secure into the soil.

- Align your spine in meditation with the tree's trunk.

- Place your bare feet on the earth, and find your ground, drop energetic roots into the soil like a tree.

Fire

Fire represents the heart, the color red, the south, high noon, summer, growth, and joy. Fire invites us to relate to creation and destruction. Our ancestors all over the globe evolved with the harnessing of fire.

It must have been through lightning strikes causing forest fires that we were first exposed to live fires other than the heat from the sun and the eruptions of volcanoes. Our early human ancestors would likely collect fire from wildfires. Many tribes all over the world learned ways to keep embers and carry them along their travels, being able to start fires for warmth and cooking. Before the advent of fire making our ancestors relied on shivering and communal sleeping for warmth.

To balance fire:

- Spend time with fire.

- Learn how to make fire, how to stoke it from scratch, how to billow it with your breath.

- Face the south and pray to the fire within and in the center of the earth, its volcanoes, and to the great sun; the embodiment of Yang energy.

Fire medicine

Do you see how fire consumes and creates? How can you build heat in your body? Utilizing hyper-oxygenating breath patterns and fast movements, a fire inside is ignited.

Tibetan monks practice Tumo, a practice of breathwork used for creating an inner fire. These monks are known for melting the snow around them when sitting in meditation.

Fire exercises:

- Meditate with a candle burning or in front of a campfire. Fixate upon the dancing flames, observe them.

- Mimic fire's movements and dance. Express your joy and bliss.

- Receive the heat, reflect on how it nourishes you.

- Notice what potential it ignites within and what it helps burn away that does not serve.

- After the fire burns away that which is not needed; say, "May new myths sprout, blowing to the wind."

Sun medicine

The human body has evolved with the rising and setting of the sun. When the eyes take in early morning sunlight, a signal is sent to the brain that it is time to wake up and when the light dims after sunset, we are signaled towards a time to sleep. This is called Circadian Rhythm. Being exposed to excess blue light, which comes from screens and synthetic light bulbs misleads our brains to believe that it's time to wake up again, especially at night.

As part of the lifestyle shift that I encourage in Elemental Embodiment, is to start every day by receiving morning light in the eyes, preferably before 9 a.m. and within an hour of waking. This morning light is a healthy dose of infrared rays.

Sun exercises:

- Within an hour of waking, before 9 a.m., expose yourself to the sunshine for 5 to 20 minutes.

- Receive the kiss of the sun, the fire in the sky, the life-giving light that is responsible for all life to exist.

- Absorb the light and turn it into Vitamin D, like how plants photosynthesize.

Metal

Metal represents the lungs and large intestine, the west, the setting sun, autumn, grief and sadness. Metal invites us to relate to what is sharp and penetrating. It is the element of the minerals created under the pressure of the earth.

To balance metal:

- Go to the wild places where crystals and metals twinkle in the darkness of caves and bestow their healing properties.

- Practice bringing consciousness to your breath and refer to the other two chapters in this book on breath: chapter 4 by Keaton and chapter 16 by Yotam.

Water

Water represents the kidneys, the north, midnight, winter, death, and fear. I make sure to drink quality water. Seek out living water that has naturally occurring minerals. City water is stripped of the good stuff and poisoned with fluoride and chlorine. I make it a point to only drink spring water.

To balance water:

- Go swimming in the ocean, lakes, or rivers and do cold plunges. Feel the soothing and the invigoration of water.

- Mediate around waterfalls and reflect upon the surge of waterways. Reflect upon what is dying within your being, what is ready to be let go of. Offer your fears to the water.

- If you live in the city and don't have access to artesian springs, then get a good water filter. Then add trace minerals or electrolytes to the water. Activate the water by swirling the cup, structuring the water molecules, and speak a prayer into it encouraging the molecules to crystallize, carrying the intention into your cells.

Water medicine

Ten minutes in the heat and then a couple of minutes in the cold. Back and forth, the heat causes vasodilation, dilating the vascular pathways, and encouraging the blood and lymph to circulate. Then the cold causes vasoconstriction and shocks the nervous system. By using contrast therapy, alternating hot and cold, the lymph pathways dilate and contract, causing a pumping of stagnant fluid aiding in reducing inflammation and detoxing systems. A unique alteration to the consciousness is achieved through this practice, inducing a meditative state.

Hot Springs are a medicine from the deep earth that we can utilize for our bodies' healing and soothing of stressors. Receive the heat, feel a deep relaxation, and thank the minerals for their activation of the different systems of the body. Bathing cultures from around the globe have communed with these natural resources from time memoriam.

Growing up around the Hot Springs of Esalen Institute, I was introduced to contrast therapy from an early age. Perched on the cliffs of Big Sur soaking in the mineral-rich geothermal waters steaming up from deep veins in the earth, I have an early fondness for balancing that ancient heat with the cool of the stream water pouring out of Hot Springs Creek in Esalen, Big Sur.

I start most days with a cold shower or a plunge into a local swimming hole. I crave the cold as it balances the heat in my body, the inflammation that I have accumulate from the physical work I do and the lifestyle choices I make. After the cold, I regulate my core temperature through movement and breath.

It is a challenging experience to do a cold practice first thing in the morning. Meeting that resistance and overcoming it makes daily tasks throughout the day more easeful. Dropping the skin temperature to 65 degrees for about five minutes induces the release of life-preserving hormones.

I advocate immersion into natural bodies of water for the deepening of connection with nature. I salute Wim Hof for his achievements in pushing the limits of cold-water immersion. He speaks about treating the cold as a teacher and a friend. Most people when they enter cold water, experience a cold shock response which causes hyperventilation. When cultivating a cold practice, it is essential to exercise breath control and focus on breathing as slowly as possible. Still the panic through your breath.

In this modern era, humans have an over-accessibility to dopamine. For example, stimulants, checking notifications on devices, and consuming sugar are ways we get short spikes in dopamine but then crash quickly.

Cold water immersion positively spikes our dopamine by around 300 percent and is said to be sustained for five to twenty-four hours, with no crashes. Positive dopamine spikes are also achieved by spending time in nature.

Water exercise:

- Start your day with 30 deep breaths and then take a cold shower or jump into a river or body of cold water.

- Go to the waterways and breathe in activated ions of the air that carry vapor from waterfalls.

- Take a sip of water and be hydrated, connect with all the varying bodies of water on this planet.

Earth

Earth represents the stomach, digestion, and the center point of the directions. The Element of earth invites us to the ground.

Remember again that you are a product of the earth, you are one with all things. Meditate into the center point of the Earth and feel your center below your navel. Whenever you feel lost or ungrounded, align to your center and the Earth's center and feel at home. You are the living embodiment of all those who came before, all of the ancestors. They have all returned to the earth, so by connecting to her you can invoke and embody your ancestors.

To balance earth:

- Seek out the wild places that are untouched by society; places where the ecosystem is intact.

- Meditate seated, lying down, or standing bare foot. Fill your body with the electrons of the earth. Feel the support from below, the unconditional love that Mother Earth has for each one of its creations.

Embodied activism

This practice of Elemental Embodiment is the embodied activism that I spoke about above. It has the potential to create harmony within the soma, the body, as well as our human relationship with the Earth and all of its elements. Again, there is a great need for this rekindling of connection with nature for creating right relation and reaching your potential.

It is my hope that you can glean what most resonates for you from my invitations here. May these practices ignite and deepen your individual human potential and inspire others whom you have a destiny with, creating a community around healing our connection with the natural world.

We must re-wild as a human society, and that starts with you. These practices can be conceptualized, though it is in *embodied remembering* what our ancestors knew and us consciously reclaiming the forgotten knowledge and kinesthetic sense, that is laden in our DNA.

"A great teacher doesn't tell us what to do; a great teacher helps us to remember that which we already know," says my teacher Tihikpas Rudolph Procter.

> *Earth my body, Water my blood,*
> *Air my breath, and Fire my Spirit.*
> — Anonymous

Let us rekindle the ancient flame within and awaken the primal song of our souls.

My prayer for you

In unity, we remember our place in the circle of life, healing the bond between humanity and the Earth.

With each breath, may we draw strength from the Earth beneath our feet.

With each step, may we walk gently upon this sacred ground, honoring all that sustains us.

May our hearts be open to the teachings of the natural world, as we strive to live in harmony and balance.

In this journey of re-wilding, may we find our true selves and inspire others to join us in this sacred mission.

Key takeaways to implement

* Incorporate prayer and gratitude:

   Learn from indigenous cultures by speaking to the land, express-ing gratitude, and relating to elements as Grandmother Earth and Grandfather Sky to foster reciprocity.

* Practice Elemental Embodiment:

   Consciously connect to the source of all life by invoking the key ingredients of earth, water, air, fire, and metal, understanding that we are made of these elements.

   Deepen connection with specific elements through practice:

   ◇ Wood: Stand among trees, look into greens, reflect on birth, scream to release anger.

   ◇ Fire: Spend time with fire, learn to make/stoke it, meditate with flames, mimic fire's movements, and practice hyper-oxygenating breathwork (like Tumo).

   ◇ Metal: Seek wild places with crystals/metals, and bring con-sciousness to your breath.

   ◇ Water: Drink quality spring water, swim in natural bodies of water, do cold plunges, meditate around waterfalls, and practice contrast therapy (alternating hot and cold).

   ◇ Earth: Seek untouched wild places, walk barefoot, and feel the support from the earth.

* Practice hormesis:

   Challenge your body with elemental stressors (like cold exposure) to reignite genetic pathways for healing and resilience, producing beneficial chemicals and hormones.

* Attune to natural cycles:

  Align your activities with the cycles of the moon and the change of seasons to cultivate well-being in body, mind, and spirit.

* Recognize embodied activism:

  Understand that your personal practice of Elemental Embodiment is a form of activism that contributes to creating harmony within yourself and healing the human relationship with the Earth.

About the author

Mac Murphy is an Esalen® Massage Therapist and Embodiment Facilitator. He grew up in Mill Valley, just north of San Francisco, among the redwood ridges and beaches surrounding Mt. Tamalpais. Mac is a fourth-generation steward of the land of The Esalen Institute in Big Sur, CA. Between the two places he has fallen in love with the magic of nature.

There is a pristine rawness of nature at Esalen. An ancient ground with a profound human history dating back 10,000 years when the Esselen People first arrived there at the end of the last Ice Age. The powerful energy of the land lives inside of him.

He is a Murphy Family representative in the healing and reconciliation efforts between the Esalen Institute and The Esselen Tribe of Monterey County. Having grown up within the Esalen community, he has had many teachers who are the original curators of the Human Potential Movement.

www.macmurphy.co

Hi, I am Chandra, the organizer and momma to this book project. It is a dream of mine, since I was a child, to write a book. My other deep passion is growth, both my own personal growth and supporting others in their own growth.

As one of my dear teachers says, "You are like the pit crew for the transformation team — you are here to help tune up bodies and brains so that human consciousness continues to evolve and expand."

— *Book momma Chandra*

10

Mood Before Food

Chandra Zas

In a world overflowing with quick fixes and symptom management, I want to share a different approach with you: relationship-based tools for lasting conscious change.

This means treating health as an ongoing, alive, and rewarding relationship you can cultivate with your body, brain, food, mood, time, stress, and above all your conscious *self*. The simple act of placing your hand on your heart and taking a slow deep breath is a form of relationship-based change.

At its essence, relationship is your thoughts and feelings — the very place where lasting transformation occurs.

The most powerful medicine lies within your mind's awareness and understanding of the signals of your own body.

- If your breathing is shallow, take it as a signal to tune in, touch your heart, breathe, and feel.

- If you are forcing a "healthy" smoothie down your throat, inquire and wonder if your body is saying no to something you think is healthy, but your body is saying otherwise.

- If you talk negatively to yourself and are feeling badly, know that you can catch and correct the thoughts in your mind to be more kind with yourself.

This is the deepest and most effective path to change because when you transform what you think and feel (your relationship) about any aspect of your life, you create conscious shifts that ripple within you and throughout your life. For example, shifting from thinking I have to exercise (which creates tension), to I want to move my body (which creates motivation) changes your physiological relationship with physical exercise.

Each thought you think (consciously or not), emotion you feel (or suppress), behavior you engage (or neglect), and even each bite you take creates a cascade of biochemical reactions. These reactions shape you: your well-being, your energy, and your experience of your life. When your internal relationships are unconscious — when you're living in tension and stress rather than in alignment with your*self*— you experience the consequences such as fatigue, mood swings, reactivity, cravings, digestive issues, and chronic health problems.

All disease starts at the emotional level.
— *Julie North*

But here's the useful truth: while you can't control what happens to you in your life, you can choose how you relate to the events in your life. You can't control your genes — but you can impact the expression of your genes by your conscious lifestyle — the root of how you show up in your life and what you create. By engaging your inner awareness and making conscious choices, you change your physiological and energetic environment.

The ripple effects of this conscious relationship extend far beyond physical health. When you invest in your inner relationships, you free up enormous mental, physical, and emotional energy. You stop battling internally and start collaborating with your innate wisdom. This relief allows you to show up resilient, resourced, and graceful in every area of your life.

I'm passionate about sharing my relationship-based approach because I've lived on both sides of it. I know the limitations of health issues and symptom management. And I know the impact of feeling healthy and symptom free. The path between these two experiences isn't quick fixes, medications, or rules — it's eating clean and regulating your stress through conscious internal relationships.

I invite you to consider: What if *the* solution you've been seeking isn't about finding the magic pill? What if it's about transforming your internal relationships? What if your health puzzle lies in you consciously relating to your thoughts and feelings? This perspective shift is the key to your new baseline of health.

My journey to relationship-based health

You have the inner ability to radically change your relationship to yourself and in the process unlock your own health puzzle. I know because I have been there and come out the other side. I have gone from not loving myself emotionally and physically, to the point of avoiding mirrors and window reflections, to wholeheartedly smiling at Me in mirrors and in window reflections.

At the age of two, I was going to specialists because I was covered head to toe in "the itches," also known as eczema; I had a long list of food allergies and asthma. I was doing biofeedback and on elimination diets when they were considered to be on the fringe of treatment. I was an unusually unwell child, dependent on several medications to deal with symptoms that created more symptoms.

As a teenager, I saw a limited and gray life ahead of me. I was overweight, constipated, and had chronic headaches; I also struggled mentally and emotionally with body image and depression. I questioned if I would ever be able to travel or have kids. I remember walking out of my doctor's office at age 15, feeling determined to find an alternative way to live a vibrant life. But I had no idea how.

My first big breakthrough came through food. After a two-week food experiment, I experienced firsthand how food impacted both my mood and my symptoms. But it was not until my 20s when I learned tools for my emotions that my understanding of food's effects on my body and brain became doable to stick to. I thought I was unusually sensitive — but when friends and friends of friends started asking for health advice, I saw that what worked for me also worked for them and their different symptoms.

This is when I realized my journey was repeatable and needed to be shared. I have deep frustration with America's medical and insurance systems because I have come to see that they are for profit and not for the people's health. If I had accepted my childhood doctor's words, that my symptoms were something to simply accept, then I wouldn't have sought out alternatives. I once felt cursed by my health but now feel blessed by the childhood health struggle that pushed me to take ownership of my health. If you are struggling with your health — then I want the same for you. My determination to figure out my health came from thinking: *I will find a way.*

The connection between body, brain, food, mood, time, and self isn't separate; it's a dynamic relationship that you can consciously elevate and use to your advantage.

Making food changes, at the root cause, means addressing your relationship — your thoughts and feelings around food. There is a pattern between feelings, food, and emotional eating: over-using food to soothe uncomfortable emotions. Food is soothing, but if overused for emotions, it creates physical havoc. When you address your relationship with your emotions first, then that relieves the need for emotional eating, which opens the doorway for a cleaner relationship with food.

Imagine creating an internal path that nourishes how you want to feel in your body and life. Picture your *self* regularly choosing, throughout each part of your day, how you want your future self to feel.

Use your mind, don't let it use you.
                                      — David

Mood-before-food

Awareness itself has the power to transform your relationship with food. As an example, learning to read ingredients and educating yourself about which ingredients your body uses for nourishment vs which ingredients your body struggles to process. Another example is keeping a food and mood journal to learn which foods energize you, vs which ingredients slow you down. Your food and mood journal can also bring awareness to why you are eating — noticing if your reason is to soothe an emotion. When you attempt to manage your emotions through comfort eating, you are band-aiding your emotional pain by pacifying it instead of processing it. The habitual connection between your mood states and eating behaviors can feel overpowering — but gaining awareness gives you the key to consciously change it.

If you are over-using food to cope and self-soothe, I encourage you to begin by identifying the emotions or stressors in your day and the go-to habits that follow, like food choices. The root cause shift won't come from the common use of judgment or discipline; it's about gaining tools for emotional regulation and working with yourself. The human brain has evolved to seek comfort and avoid pain (including emotional pain) by coping with a variety of pacifiers like eating, drinking, or scrolling. The key is finding natural and beneficial options instead of costly quick fixes. For example, spending time in nature while leaning in and feeling vs scrolling and avoiding feeling.

It doesn't matter how clean you eat if you are stressed.
                                      — Erin Sharman ND

If you want to reach your health potential, then you need to do the inner work of creating a conscious relationship with your emotions.

I encourage you to befriend your emotions; let them be in a metaphorical car with you — but you stay in the driver seat. You choose when and why you go to the fridge; doing so will create new neural pathways that will support you physiologically and habit-wise. When your relationship with your emotions opens, food shifts happen naturally.

Instead of forcing your *self* to eat "healthy," befriend your body's signals and underlying emotions.

I used to have a binging problem; I didn't realize all the stressors in my life. Getting to the root cause is where it's at.
— Donna

The mood-before-food approach emphasizes that your emotional state directly impacts you physiologically and your habit choices: your digestive system, hormones, inflammation, and nutrient absorption, along with your inner availability to consciously choose quality habits like food choices. When you're stressed, your body diverts energy away from digestion, leading to poor nutrient absorption and increased inflammation. When you are in emotional pain your brain urges you to *self*-soothe. By addressing the emotional component first (with high quality self-soothing), you create physiological conditions for optimal nourishment — physically and emotionally.

Instead of restricting your food choices, create a kind relationship with your future self that is focused on how you want to feel after your meal. You can do this by working consciously with your thoughts and your emotions. For example, when you shift what you unconsciously think about your emotions (from *I shouldn't feel this* to *this feeling is part of my human experience*), you shift your emotions from resistance to acceptance. Doing this internal practice will both lower your physiological stress and reduce your urge to emotionally eat — allowing food to be what it's meant to be: nourishment rather than emotional soothing.

The practice begins with awareness. Notice the emotions that precede your food choices. Invoke curiosity and acceptance. For anxiety, get curious about what emotion you're resisting or avoiding; consider some intentional breathing or a short walk with reflection and feeling. For frustration, notice what your brain is thinking that *shouldn't be happening* and notice what you are angry about. Address and tend to both what you want and the unconscious expectation your brain has. Frustration is a mix of anger and thinking, *It shouldn't be this way.*

As you engage internally with curiosity and awareness, you create internal space for new habits; food naturally shifts from being an emotional crutch to being a source of energy. You'll start ease-fully making food choices based on what your body truly needs rather than what your emotions need for coping.

This is where your empowered and aligned relationship with your health lies — in the space between emotion and action. You have the option to notice your feelings (and tend to them) without being controlled by them. You possess the inner ability to pause and to choose your response rather than react automatically. This internal relationship upgrade creates your vitality, well-being, and lasting conscious change on all levels.

From conventional to holistic

For the last 100 years, the conventional western medicine approach has focused on one part of the human body at a time, providing symptom management and for-the-average-person health recommendations. But this approach often misses a person's unique genes, personal life's circumstances, and even body signals.

Holistic medicine offers a more nuanced, interconnected, and personal approach — one where you can learn your body's unique needs, make personal lifestyle shifts to re-balance, and gain *self*-health knowledge to heal and thrive. In this nuanced holistic approach, you are an interconnected physical, mental, emotional, and spiritual *being*. When you step into honoring the messages from your body, mind, heart, and soul then the messages become contributing information, that *all* together co-create your well-being.

Positioning your*self* here, in a place of internal honoring and *self*-referencing, puts you in control of your own health potential.

During my studies of Ayurveda, an ancient Indian approach to medicine, I studied how to read a person's pulse on their wrist. Feeling beneath my fingertips the energies of their systems, including emotional, physical, and mental. I witnessed and applied a new understanding of health as a multitude of inner systems that we can shift and rebalance from many angles. For example, food affects inflammation in the body and so does stress, each angle can be addressed. This study transformed my own journey. For example, I found that by addressing my avoidant relationship to my emotions, I could lower my emotional stress. This shift rippled into my food choices from pacifying to nourishing.

This holistic approach acknowledges that all the parts of you contain signals to be addressed and tended to. Rather than taking a pill for a symptom, you can relearn to listen and rebalance yourself by honoring your internal signals. This creates an aligned rather than compartmentalized relationship within you — one that supports your expanded consciousness.

Beyond food

This use of relationship-based change extends beyond food. It encompasses anything that feels stressful to you, like time, work, friends, family, parenting, money, and/or making decisions. You can apply this conscious relationship to any given topic.

For example, when you shift what you think and feel about:

- time (from there's never enough, to I have what I need),

- work (from it is draining, to it provides money for my life),

- and relationships (from they should behave differently, to they are who they are), you are changing your physiological stress levels, your emotional state, and your access to higher level habits. Tending to these areas of your life at the relationship level makes stress and tensions melt which allows vitality to flow.

Your experience in this process will become kind of addictive — in a good way. You get to choose how you *want* to feel. You gain access to deciding how you consciously frame your experience: as a stressful event or part of your human experience. You'll feel better and you will want more.

Get hooked on good mood food: Food reset

I invite you to experience firsthand how quickly your body can recalibrate when you give it a chance. Even most "healthy" labeled foods is trickster marketing — processed products designed to trigger dopamine and boost sales rather than nourish your body and brain.

Try this: For 14 days, focus on bringing in foods that satisfy your body's true cravings. Eat only whole, single-ingredient foods: eat organic foods ideally. This simple experiment creates a profound reset in your taste buds, dopamine pathways, microbiome, and natural cravings.

Within days, you'll notice your palate becoming more sensitive to the natural sweetness in fruits and vegetables. Foods you once found bland will reveal complex, satisfying flavors. The dopamine-driven cravings for hyperpalatable processed foods will diminish as your brain resets its reward pathways to appreciate whole food. Upping your proteins and fats will reduce sugar and carb cravings physiologically.

Instead of the default of food restriction — imagine discovery through relationship experimentation. Make your thoughts and feelings about food *conscious.* As you shift from thinking, *I can't have foods I love,* to *I wonder how I will feel if I eat more whole food,* you also shift from feeling restricted to feeling curious, which gets more of yourself on board with nourishing choices. When you approach food upgrades with curiosity, you will feel energized, which makes food changes more accessible and enjoyable.

By bringing in food that satisfy the cells of your body, you liberate your body's natural ability to recognize and crave what serves your body and brain. This is the most effective way to create lasting change — through a relationship based on curiosity and true craving nourishment.

The beauty of this food reset is its simplicity and the immediate feedback your body provides. No complicated rules or calculations, just real food, intentional curiosity, and your body's remarkable ability to respond when given the chance. This direct experience will teach you how much food impacts you and will help you develop a preference for foods that make you feel good.

Create an intentional relationship with time

Are you living in a constant state of not enough time and too much to do? Are you feeling perpetually behind, rushed, busy, and/or overwhelmed? This low-level relationship with time impacts your stress levels, digestive system, immune function, hormones, food choices, and brain's ability to make quality decisions.

Creating an intentional relationship with time is an essential component of emotional regulation, lowering physiological stress, and living at your potential. Instead of cramming more into each day—or checking out altogether—create a conscious relationship with your time by deciding your priorities in advance and focusing on what matters most to you. I encourage you to start with your free time, social time, and self-care time.

The first step is to become aware of your current relationship with time and notice the costs. What are your thoughts and feelings about how you use your time? Do you feel overwhelmed? Are you perpetually thinking, *I have too much to do?* Do you multitask to the point of not being fully present? Do you find your*self* making rushed low-level decisions that cost you in mistakes and don't align with your priorities?

Next, practice making decisions about your use of your time, ahead of time. When you decide in advance how you want to spend your time — you reduce the number of low-level decisions throughout your day. This helps remedy the exhaustion that comes from rushing around and trying to do it all.

You can't do it all; you can do what matters most to you.

This intentional approach to time allows you to align your actions with your priorities rather than reacting to whatever seems most urgent in the moment. For example, deciding ahead of time that stocking the fridge with nourishing food for the week will set your *self* up to be less likely to reach for convenient but less nourishing options when you're hungry and tired. Same goes for kid or social-time: how much quality, fully present time do you want to spend? Stop feeling guilty about not spending enough time by deciding ahead of time, consciously. The same goes for your to-do list: look at what unnecessary to-dos can be crossed off when your regulated nervous system is a top priority.

I made a pact with myself. I decided that there is almost nothing worth rushing for. Going to the ER is the only time that I am willing to rush; everything else, I focus on keeping myself physiologically regulated. I invite you to bring your attention to what the feeling of rushing, stress, or urgency feels in like in your body, then consider if the physiological stress is worth it to you or not.

Quality presence
When you make decisions ahead of time, you not only will have lower stress levels, but you will also experience a heightened level of presence and satisfaction. When you're eating, focus entirely on eating — notice the flavors, textures, and signals from your body. When you're moving,

be present in your movement — feel your muscles, your breath, your energy. This presence not only enhances your mood but also improves digestion, nutrient absorption, productivity, energy levels, decision-making, and overall well-being.

Learning to manage my time and energy efficiently was significant. I learned to be clear about how I want to use my time and be present in each activity. This has been life-changing for me.

— Val

When you transform your relationship with time from one of rushing, overwhelm, or stress to one of intentionality and presence, you create the conditions for vibrant health on every level. Your nervous system can relax, your digestion improves, your energy increases, and you make food choices based on what truly nourishes you rather than what's quickest, most convenient, or has the biggest dopamine hit.

This shift in your relationship with time isn't about doing more — it's about aligning your use of time with your conscious wants and priorities, including a well-regulated nervous system. It's about quality rather than quantity, presence rather than trying to do it all. Awareness and intention are key.

Building your personalized path

Your health, your vitality, your life experience — it all begins and transcends with cultivating a conscious relationship with your thoughts and feelings. This is your most powerful tool for conscious change, and it's always available to you.

Create a "listening for" and "honoring of" your internal relationships. Consider and adjust to your unique biochemistry, genes, circumstances, and conscious wants.

First, clarify how you want to feel: energetic, calm, strong, present, and clear-minded. These desired feelings become your compass for decisions about food, time, movement, rest, and stress management.

Next, assess your current patterns without judgment, simply gathering information about what supports or detracts from your desired emotional state. From there, reverse engineer small, sustainable shifts that respect your current reality while moving you toward your goals.

As these changes become your new normal, build upon them gradually based on your desire. This approach allows for true embodiment rather than temporary compliance commonly followed by *self*-sabotage. Throughout this process, remain curious, adjusting based on your internal cues rather than rigid adherence to a plan.

Improvements in one area create positive ripple effects in others. Cleaner food ingredients lead to improved mood and mental clarity. Reduced stress improves digestion and decision making. Emotional processing supports better food choices and increased presence. By tending to your whole *self*, you create aligned effects that nourish your potential.

The result is a way of living that supports a baseline of vitality — moving through life with clarity about what serves you, ease in making beneficial choices, and integrity in your relationship with your *self*. It is not about perfection but about consciousness and presence, creating internal relationships that support the vibrant, alive version of *you*.

Key takeaways to implement

* Start with simple relationship-based awareness:

  ⬦ Bring your awareness to your thoughts and feelings.

  ⬦ Notice how different foods affect your energy and mood.

  ⬦ Observe the thoughts and feelings that drive your eating decisions.

  ⬦ Pay attention to how your emotional state influences your coping choices.

  ⬦ Consider ahead of time what your priorities are and make a plan to focus your time there with the help of connecting to your future self.

* Practice pausing between emotion and action:

  When you notice an urge to emotionally cope with food, pause for 10 seconds. During this brief window, put your hand on your heart, take three deep breaths, name the emotion you're feeling, and ask your*self* what you truly need in this moment and how you want to feel an hour from now. This simple practice interrupts automatic patterns and creates space for conscious choice, allowing you to respond to your emotional needs directly rather than using food to cope.

* Implement mindful transition moments:

  Identify three daily transition moments (like waking up, arriving home, before meals) and use them as opportunities to pause and reconnect with yourself. During each transition, put your hand on your heart, take three conscious breaths and ask: *How do I want to feel in the next part of my day?*

  This practice interrupts autopilot patterns and creates multiple opportunities throughout the day to make conscious, connected choices.

From there, continue to expand and upgrade your habits from a state of consciousness and curiosity.

Remember that this journey isn't about doing it right — it's about doing what is aligned within you and choosing consciously. Each moment offers you a new opportunity to choose relationship over rules, nourishment over restriction, and alignment over resistance.

Your thoughts and feelings are the internal relationship you can start to shift today that will enhance the rest of your life. By choosing to relate differently to your body, your brain, your food, your emotions, and your conscious *self,* you set in motion a cascade of positive changes that extend far beyond today. This is your power. This is your path. This is your potential.

About the author

Chandra specializes in relationship-based change, helping people transform their connections with stress, food, mood, time, and themselves. Her journey from a chronically ill child covered in eczema and dependent on prescription medications to a vibrant guide for transformation began with a pivotal food experiment at age fifteen that allowed her to "feel the difference." This breakthrough led to five years of intensive study at Esalen Institute and BodyMind Restoration retreats, where she developed her signature "Mood Before Food" philosophy – understanding that lasting change requires addressing emotional relationships before dietary shifts actually stick.

Chandra brings together diverse approaches to growth through consciousness and transformation. Her work extends beyond individual healing to what she sees as the "transformation team" – people committed to helping humanity evolve and grow. Through her programs, she guides parents, entrepreneurs, and grandparents through yearlong consciousness journeys that address the root causes of disconnection rather than managing symptoms. Her approach integrates ancient wisdom with modern understanding, recognizing that our relationship with stress, emotions, and unconscious patterns directly impacts our health, life experience, and potential.

Chandra's mission centers on empowering people to become their own health advocates, developing the internal tools necessary for sustainable transformation. Living in Reno with her husband and daughter, she practices what she teaches through radical parenting that honors children's inner wisdom and body signals. Her work demonstrates that when we heal our relationship with ourselves – learning to listen to our bodies, manage our time and life stressors consciously, and gain internal awareness – we create ripple effects that extend far beyond personal health to impact families, communities, and future generations. She believes that true healing happens not through restriction and rules, but through curiosity, consciousness, and coming home to ourselves.

Learn more about Chandra's work, offerings, and philosophy at:

chandrazas.com

@ChandraZas

Part Four

Brain Changers for Healing

Jim coaches in Carhartts, approaching trauma recovery with both serious dedication and healing laughter. His book, *Wounds to Wisdom*, outlines his effective methodology for overcoming trauma's grip on life and transforming painful experiences into sources of strength and insight.

Jim's work shows that the cycle of intergenerational pain can stop with each of us when we commit to healing ourselves.

— *Book momma Chandra*

11

Heal Deep Trauma to Create an Alive Life

Jim Pehkonen

There are wounds that never show on the body that
are deeper and more hurtful than anything that bleeds.
— Laurell K. Hamilton

Reaching your highest level of human potential is your birthright. Yet trauma tends to create the mental space within you that may hinder you from being your best. As a coach who focuses on trauma, I will share with you: the impact of trauma and how it limits your potential, I'll introduce you to the first step of processing trauma, and how you can begin to step into your highest potential through trauma work.

Mental health since 2020 has shifted. The trauma associated with the pandemic has created higher cases of suicide, addiction, and depression. With many people in isolation, stress and fear, the impact on mental health has been harsh and real. Out of this event, humanity will be recovering for years, maybe decades. There are steps to adjust to this new life through much needed trauma work, resulting in the potential of a better life through healing. This potential is now buried deeper in the pile of trauma. Yet it is there.

Every human experiences a level of trauma as they grow up in this world. Each person is impacted in various degrees by their experience of trauma before the age of five. No one is immune. NO ONE! Yet, in my work over the last 20 years as a coach, I have made a unique observation and created the space for my clients, through their work, to step into their greatest human potential by assisting them to understand how they create this reality we call life. I have written a book based on my almost 20 years of coaching that is focused on trauma processing and the healing that can occur called *Wounds to Wisdom: The Art of Healing Trauma*.

Some people seem to have a natural ability to grow and succeed in spite of their early life traumas, yet others suffer greatly the older they get. Far more people's lives are seriously impacted at times by what would appear to be a typical trauma. As this trauma has become the *baseline* by which they create their experience of life, it operates within their consciousness undetected until they do the work to understand the original baseline trauma or break from love, and its impact on how they have created their life up to this point.

Your "break from love" impact

When I talk about "love" in my work, it is the space each human is born into inside their heart. A newborn simply has a space of being that is "love" and also, when not in that space, is in a space that I call "not-of-love." These are the original two spaces each young human is born into. As each human experiences more in the world, "Love" and "not-of-love" get expanded out as a result of life experiences, which create all the emotional states that people experience in life.

Understanding it was the breaks from that initial love you were born out of and into. Your life has been filled with the most incredible moments, as well as the shadow moments of darkness. As a result of the trauma, traditional societal responses to certain behaviors and emotional states push you toward pharmaceuticals and ongoing therapeutic interventions as opposed to deepening your understanding of how your human experience is created. The more you understand your mind, mindset, and how you create this incredible thing called life, the fewer pharmaceuticals and therapeutic time you will need to spend on yourself.

Let's look for a moment at the traditional therapeutic and pharmaceutical model. Neither creates the space of long-lasting healing, they simply are not healing-driven. Once you are diagnosed and the right pills have been tested and physically stabilized, you stay on these pharmaceuticals for life. And in so many cases, your world loses the peaks and valleys and simply becomes almost a flat line of numbness and basic survival.

Most therapeutic training and licensing set up the space where your life cannot be handled without that weekly visit to your therapist. These visits mostly have you learn to deal with the impact of your trauma in your mind in a way that tolerates the trauma yet never really heals anything. "How was your last week?" is often the first question that leads endless sessions of toleration; because what it asks is: *How are you relating to life with your trauma since the last visit?* You talk through your weekly mindset until the session is over and then set up the next weekly appointment.

Over the years, I have had numerous clients who had more than 10 years of traditional therapy. In one instance, a previous client had 18 years of therapy. Through our work, in under two years, she was able to understand and transform her life and now lives an incredible life.

Now, there is a time and place for pharmaceuticals and therapy, yet if you have been in therapy for more than four years, you may find your visits are simply how you deal with your trauma since the last visit, instead of doing the deep work to actually truly heal yourself and begin to step into living fully in an amazing life. Pharmaceuticals and therapy have a time and place but often neglect the root cause; therefore, I believe getting to your break from "not-of-love" is the best place to turn when mental behavior shifts into the negative.

Let me share my experience of the coaching I do. It is about helping my clients transform their experience of the life they create. Most clients coach with me for about 12 months unless the level of trauma is such that longer work is needed. The deeper their understanding of their experience — the more they can process their story and the impact of their trauma; ultimately shifting their experience of living.

My clients learn to experience the joys and wonders in the world while also being able to experience the sadness, pain, and low points in life. They create a world where the highs and the lows happen, and they powerfully deal with the exact place they are. They create a life they believe and feel is worth living. In order to get here, both my clients and you first need to understand this concept called trauma.

The concept of trauma

Every human who walks this planet has suffered a level of trauma. Mostly, it happens early in life, and then we literally create an experience of life based on the reaction to early trauma. Through understanding, you can stop the suffering and create a new experience of life.

There is an art to healing trauma. My mission in life is to assist people to heal from the ghosts of their past.

Life today has developed the perception of instant healing, yet the truth is that understanding the process required to step into an incredible life takes intentional work. Authentic and direct work so you can begin to understand how the events of your childhood have created who you are as you begin this work. Yet, in doing this work, you open up the potential to shift the direction of life.

If traditional methods of dealing with your drama and trauma have not worked, this may be the perfect time to see if an alternative method might be the thing that allows you to step into your healing.

As you begin this unique healing journey, let's define what trauma is. My definition of trauma is: your emotional response to an event that occurred, which lives on in your mind and creates a state of mental 'not-of-love'. Trauma creates a long-term impact on your mental, emotional, and physical well-being.

You have the power within you. Yet events in your life have created the space where this power may not seem real, and the "demons" inside seem more powerful than the light inside of you. It's time to begin to understand the impact of these mental wounds to the point where *you* do the work required to create an incredible life!

So, let's look at you for a moment. What is the lens through which you see life? Are you willing to deepen the understanding of that which has slowed you, hindered you, and, in some cases, stopped you from living an amazing life?

As you go through these exercises, I have a few requests:

- Go gentle on yourself through the work.

- Choose to love yourself for doing this work.

- Know that there will be good and bad days, as a wise person once told me about every moment: *This too shall pass.*

- Create a support network of people who have been there for you and have them agree to be your support team through your growth.

So, let's begin. Your growth awaits you!

Exercise #1: Documentation of your healing journey

As you begin this healing adventure, my request is you document your transformation. This may be either by journaling and or taking a video of yourself as you are in this current moment and ongoing as you transform yourself. In documentation, you will tell yourself how you are, the impact of the trauma, and how life is through this journey. This gets to be the measure of your transformation.

For your documentation, find a space and place to do the work. Answer the following as a minimum. Feel free to add more as you see fit. This is for you and your growth. Talk about where you are in life as you begin this journey. Some things to potentially address:

- Your name

- Your struggle

- Where you are in life right now

- How you see life as a result of past childhood traumas

- The impact of trauma on your life today

- What you would like to achieve out of this work

- What effort are you willing to make to achieve a transformation?

- Where might you fail?

- Where might you succeed?

- Are you willing to commit to doing the exercises, even if they are challenging?

Feel free to add questions and comments as the recording happens.

Before you record, you may want to write out the above questions as a reflection of where life is for you as you begin. Save this writing. It gets to be the map of the journey you are taking. The beauty of writing and recording where you are is it gets to be the space for you to document where you are as you begin your journey. Wherever life is right now, this is the space you are in as you begin this healing journey.

This will not be easy. You may feel like it is silly, or you may not want to be so vulnerable. Yet you are far stronger than you realize. You have survived every day before this one, you have navigated this adventure called life, and now you are beginning a journey that has the potential for the most profound life transformation to date.

There are points along the journey where you will do another video journal. As you have major epiphanies, journal and do a video journal of your realizations. During your review times and when you are in a low vibrational state, these get to be the places to potentially give you hope along the way. Yes, it will be hard, and you can do the "hard exercises" in life that cause you to grow in ways you cannot fully see in this present moment.

Before you stop reading the chapter because of your potential discomfort with doing a video, let's talk about this. Taking videos of yourself can seem silly, weird, and often very unnerving. The first one will seem awkward as you describe life today. Yet when you have transformed yourself, you will watch and be able to see the progress of your hard work. Yes, you get to be vulnerable. That voice in your head will say this is really an unreasonable request.

Save these videos in a safe place. They are going to be what you use along this journey to document your growth. You can do these videos whenever you feel like recording your progress.

You will look back and be very thankful that you actually did this. Give it an attempt and see what happens. You get to create a video that shows you (and only you) how you were as you began this journey. Down the road, you will smile as you watch it. You will see just how far your growth has gone.

Exercise #2: Mapping your internal mind landscape

Healing ... you *so* have this. The first step is often the toughest. Together, we have this!

Let's go through one more exercise that assists you to reflect upon your internal landscape, now and through the process of your transformation. As you process and heal trauma, your "internal landscape" will change. There are times when drawing out a pictorial drawing to represent your "internal landscape" is very effective. Over my years of coaching, I have used a few different methods to represent someone's internal landscape. This one has been the most effective and transformational for my clients who are inclined to draw out how it "looks" inside. I initially learned it in a workshop very early in my coaching career and have modified it over the years.

I had some resistance to this when I first learned it. I have not really considered myself an artist, yet through this exercise, I was able to learn to express myself through some very simple exercises. So, you may be initially hesitant to draw your internal landscape out. My request is: do it! You may be very surprised at how it transforms you in the most wonderful manner. Let's get into your internal landscape.

What if your internal landscape could be represented by a picture you draw of a landscape? It takes some pondering and sketching and artwork. NOTE: I am probably the artist where drawing is one of my least desirable ways to express myself. I'm actually not the best artist, and if I can do this, I KNOW you can do this.

The first time I did this, I only used a pencil, sketching it up as a black-and-white drawing. Later versions, as I transformed myself, I ended up with full-color sketches. The color represented the vibrancy and life I was putting into my life.

The objective of this chapter is to begin to "see" the quality of your life through expressed art. I believe it is possible to create a "garden landscape" picture of how you "see" the quality of your life. And the trauma you have experienced in life can most certainly be a part of this landscape. It happened, and it is a part of your life experience.

Sometimes, it is easy to simply begin with a sheet of paper and begin drawing a landscape.

Some essential items:

- How does love flow through your landscape?

- Make sure you put in your favorite land features; for me, I have prairies that blow with the wind, mountains that represent

obstacles AND victories, roads between different areas of my being, pretty flowers that express growth, activities that feed my soul,
and different animals that I resonate with.

- Your early landscapes may show areas that you feel stagnant or
  stuck in. I have always placed a wellspring of love in my landscapes. In my early drawings, it did not have much flow and
  represented the wellspring of love as a swamp. As I cleared my
  heart and love began flowing again, the spring began flowing
  clear, and the resulting landscape grew and became lush again.
  Be open to your "land features" shifting as you transform yourself.

A small garden may grow to be a great garden; a grove of trees may
suddenly have a swing or treehouse appear as clarity and joy. Use bright
colors; your life will appear more vibrant and enlivened.

After a while, I could simply close my eyes and see the symbolic
representation of how I was feeling inside. I used to imagine the landscape, and over time, I learned how to increase the flow of love from my
wellspring of love, which made my landscape become very vibrant and
alive. Over time, I can "see" areas where my thinking is deteriorating the
landscape by simply imagining it. Then I go back and "see" where my
thinking is also deteriorating. It was a powerful way to understand myself
pictorially.

You also have the power of creation. What would you like your
"mind's landscape" to look like? Add those features. If you have mental
resistance, notice that this resistance is the area of growth for you. Pay
close attention to it and ask your internal being what this means for you.

As you do this a few times, you may want to journal about the items
that will make your garden more vibrant and empowered. Allow your imagination to inspire your mental landscape. Remember, at the end of the day,
this is YOUR mental landscape, and you get to say how it appears.

As a result of your first drawing, you may want to create an action
plan to take your landscape to the next level. As you transform through

your trauma, review your action plan, and draw your new landscape. Your growth gets to be reflected in your mental landscape. You are the creator of your reality, and this mental landscape gets to be the internal mirror and an external picture for reflection as evidence of your growth.

I have not included any of my drawings. You can draw up simple landscapes, and chances are yours will look far better than mine! Yours will be the reflection of how you create your internal landscape.

Internal landscape instructions

Sketch out your internal landscape. Using paper, just draw out the internal landscape of your "inner world." Here is a partial list of features:

- A spring representing love flowing into your being. For mine, this tended to be in the center and lead to a stream flowing through all areas.

- An area representing nourishment. It might be a garden or fields.

- An area representing adventure in your life. Might be a forest for exploring, a mountain with slopes for skiing, a desert for exploring, a river with adventure on the river, or maybe your favorite camping spot.

- An area representing growth in life. Draw this as you see growth.

- A bright sun representing the radiance of life that feeds the garden and other areas.

- Paths or roads connecting the different areas of your life.

- Other aspects you feel are important to be reflected in your drawing.

Do these drawings as you heal. Notice how healing in one area impacts the rest of your landscape. Even if you do this weekly, bi-weekly, or monthly, this becomes a pictorial representation of your transformation.

Now if these two exercises have made a difference for you, I have written a book called *Wounds to Wisdom: The Art of Healing Trauma* —

you can find where to buy my book at the end of my chapter. It has more in depth exercises similar to the above that take you through the process I have used over the last 18-plus years to assist people to process their past trauma and begin to live an incredible life from this day forward.

Emerging field of psychedelic trauma healing

The emerging field of using psychedelics to assist coaching is showing promise in enhancing the coaching process, particularly for individuals grappling with deep-seated emotional or psychological barriers. When administered in a controlled, therapeutic setting with trained professionals, psychedelics like psilocybin or ketamine can facilitate profound shifts in perspective, allowing people to access and process previously inaccessible memories or traumas.

This can create breakthroughs in self-awareness and emotional release, making individuals more receptive to coaching that enhances the coaching process. By addressing core issues and dismantling limiting beliefs, psychedelic experiences can clear the path for coaches to guide clients toward greater self-understanding, personal growth, and the achievement of their goals. However, it's crucial to emphasize that this is a specialized area requiring strict protocols, qualified oversight, and careful integration of the psychedelic experience with ongoing coaching support. It is not a replacement for traditional coaching, but rather a potentially powerful adjunct for specific client needs.

To learn more about the power of psychedelics, please refer to the chapter by Dr. Burton J. Tabaac and the chapter by Greg Jones in this part of our handbook. Psychedelic healing is proving to be safe and effective, within the guidelines being established for successful healing in the use of psychedelics.

Key takeaways to implement

* Exercise #1 — Documentation of your healing journey

  This is for you and your growth. Talk about where you are in life as you begin this journey.

* Exercise #2 — Mapping your internal mind landscape

  Sketch out your internal landscape. Using paper, just draw out the internal landscape of your "inner world." Do these drawings as you heal. Notice how healing in one area impacts the rest of your landscape. Even if you do this weekly, bi-weekly, or monthly, this becomes a pictorial representation of your transformation.

* Get my book *Wounds to Wisdom* to learn about alternate processes to address life trauma.

About the author

Jim Pehkonen is a Life Architect, a trained and certified Life Coach working with clients experiencing deep trauma, addiction recovery, and leadership development. With over 18 years of experience coaching in one-on-one settings and group workshops, he assists his clients in understanding how they create this experience called life. This is his life mission. His approach introduces out-of-the-box modalities to help you understand the impact of their thinking on the bottom-line results in their life. Jim's personal style is intuitive and unique. His natural coaching instinct enables his clients to rapidly achieve results.

In 2003, he began his own transformation, and during the next 10 years of intense experiential study, he healed himself first, then grew and developed a coaching business to assist others. He uses a range of healing modalities to support others in their personal transformations.

With his past experience as a General Manager in a construction company and trauma recovery coaching in addiction recovery facilities;

Jim can help people from all walks of life. This allows him to work with broken businesses to redevelop their team communication, help individuals connect with themselves, and impact family dynamics so members are able to have more peaceful relationships.

Jim currently serves on the Board of Directors for Sierra Psychedelic Society as the Community Outreach person, leading Integration Circles and supporting community education about the benefits of psychedelic use.

Realizing that the impact of one-to-one coaching and even workshops was limited to those who could attend in person; Jim stepped into writing so more people like you could be positively affected by his experience, drive, and passion.

The website associated with his latest book can be found at www.WoundsToWisdomBook.com.

Jim can be reached through his website or by email at Jim@AmazingLifeDesign.com.

AmazingLifeDesign.com

Through love, war, grief, loss, and healing Yotam has walked his talk, returning always to the simple, accessible healing power of breath. As a true medicine man offering bodywork, breathwork, acupuncture, and now written teachings, his presence itself is healing.

His chapter offers practical breathing techniques that can transform your trauma and your daily life.

— *Book momma Chandra*

12

Minimize the Lasting Impact of Pain and Suffering with Therapeutic Breathing

Yotam Tamari

I'm releasing my soul to the endless current of light and rebirthing," my best friend wrote in his journal days before he died in military service and an hour after I last spoke with him. I was conscious of my sadness. I let myself feel it. Later, I could see how it was impacting my ability to feel joy, but I accepted that. You and I both cannot stop life and the pains that come with it; you can consciously respond to and allow life's pain through your human being and body to avoid getting stuck in trauma.

Breath is the tool I want to share with you so that you can avoid getting stuck with pain and trauma in your body.

The difference between trauma and painful emotions is in how we respond to and process it. To understand that life continues to move, you and I both have the option to choose life or to remain stuck.

Human potential is using your infinite intelligence inside your body. Infinite intelligence is breaking something very complex down into something simple, using mental and physical terms to walk inside this reality with minimum suffering. This, for me, is human potential, because life is full of pain and suffering. The question is when you encounter pain and suffering — how you can minimize the lasting impact.

Understanding trauma and the nervous system

Trauma often comes from an inability to process reality — when it's too much, too fast. The body contracts, breathing becomes shallow, and emotions get stuck. That shallow breath is what locks the trauma in place.

But if you intervene, if you help someone breathe deeply in that moment, you can reverse the experience. You can bring consciousness to the breath and move the emotional energy. That's a big piece of what breathwork can offer.

Talking about trauma means talking about the autonomic nervous system, which includes both the sympathetic and parasympathetic systems. This system is what gets damaged in trauma — but it's also the key to healing that damage. There are studies that show how trauma lights up certain parts of the brain on an X-ray, compared to non-traumatized people.

Your nervous system is made of three subsystems; one of them is the autonomic nervous system. This autonomic system is divided into two parts: parasympathetic and sympathetic.

These two systems are related to fight or flight mode. The autonomic nervous system regulates all stimulation from the environment to the central nervous system. Every stimulation needs to pass a barrier where the brain says, "Okay, that's interesting information." If you touch something hot like fire, you instinctively pull your hand back because the stimulation is very strong. But if a small ant crawls on your hand, most probably you won't feel it because the stimulation is not strong enough.

When something very stressful happens, your autonomic nervous system responds by activating your sympathetic system, which creates stress. The electrical charges that fire between the brain and the organs are immense and overload the system. Your sympathetic is activated for example when a tiger chases you. Which means your sympathetic system pushes blood away from your torso into your limbs, so you have oxygen to run or fight. Your pupils expand, your hearing sharpens, and you become more alert to even the smallest stimulations, which is useful in survival situations.

How are these systems related to trauma?

When something stressful happens, the sympathetic nervous system responds, and trauma occurs when your system gets stuck in sympathetic mode. The regulation of the system depends on one another; only when the parasympathetic is stronger, then the sympathetic nervous system subdues. Breath is the best fundamental tool of the body to stimulate the parasympathetic system.

Trauma is directly related to the nervous system, specifically to these two systems. Where the parasympathetic is responsible for resting, digesting, making love, and orgasm. The sympathetic is linked to stress, running, and being alert to external threats.

When you live with chronic stress, that regulation starts to fail. The sympathetic system takes over, and the nervous system gets stuck in stress mode. One way to re-regulate and flip your system back into parasympathetic is through long exhalations. If you exhale for more than eight seconds, you can directly regulate your nervous system, regardless of your body's current state.

You don't have to wait for calm to arrive — you can create it.

I personally do breathwork that includes multiple techniques, but over time I have gotten to a place where I'm inhaling for five seconds and exhaling for 30 seconds; just two breaths a minute. That's how I regulate myself. It's not as hard as it sounds, and it gives me control over my state, no matter how much stress I'm under.

Stress can be useful, like if your kid breaks their leg and you need to rush to the hospital, that adrenaline is helpful, or you are running from a tiger. But for someone like a firefighter, or a lawyer with a high-pressure job, living in chronic stress is not useful.

Your autonomic nervous system is one-third of all the electrical charges which move inside your body. Your autonomic nervous system defines you, your energy, your emotional experiences, your communication with yourself and with your environment — your way of being in the world.

Use breath to reset

For people with really stressful lives, the key is to identify where stress feels most damaging. Some people feel stuck in the morning, they can't get going because the pressure is too overwhelming. Others feel wired at night when they should be tired.

In both cases, breath is the tool. You don't have to wait until bedtime or a yoga class. Take five minutes right in that moment, morning or night, to regulate your breath. Five minutes is enough. That small window can completely shift your state.

There was a study that looked at pranayama, the yogic breath technique, and with as little as five minutes a day it showed to have huge benefits. Better sleep, improved focus, and digestion; proof breathing physiologically works.

Emotions, fear, and your freeze response

Breathing is a window that shows you what's happening inside of you. The main cause of freezing is emotions like fear and anxiety — fear of life, fear of death, fear of pain.

When emotions come in, in Chinese medicine and in the English word, *e-motion* implies motion — movement of the feeling. So, the motion of fear and anxiety makes the emotion dissolve.

Fear without breath can make you freeze. If you can observe what's happening and say, "Okay, my best friend died," and step outside of the situation, and understand, "This is what I'm feeling now. This is what is happening." This awareness and intentional breathing make the sympathetic system begin to regulate itself.

The sympathetic and parasympathetic go together — when one rises, the other falls, and vice versa.

When you stay in motion, stay moving while experiencing difficult things in life, by overcoming the natural urge of freezing, by instead observing and breathing — you're able to the internal regulation of your nervous system and help it avoid getting stuck — avoiding an imprint of trauma on your system.

An interesting study showed that in people experiencing trauma, the areas activated in their brains are related directly to survival — eating, sleeping, and safety. No communication, no creativity, no socializing — nothing else.

This study shows the sympathetic system is stuck and not moving, correlating directly to the brain's imprint of emotional states during and after traumatic events. The longer someone waits without proper treatment after a traumatic event, the more the electrical nervous patterns become stamped in the brain, creating and hardwiring neural pathways that are very hard to unwire.

A good example is when mammals are attacked by large predators like lions. If they survive, they engage in very heavy breathing for hours afterward.

Breathing is the key that can help keep your central organ system be in motion supporting your nervous system to regulate itself.

Breathing to self-regulate

Breathing itself doesn't directly help you step out of trauma, but it's a key to sending messages that regulate the nervous system. There are more ways, but breathing is the main action you can take. For example, if someone has a car accident and immediately afterward is taken for a walk and encouraged to breathe and process, they most likely won't become stuck in trauma.

If you keep your emotions moving in life, you won't get stuck. Certainly, there's a lot to address, treat, and discuss, but the nervous system will remain intact.

A traumatic event does not *have* to create trauma in a person's body, brain, and nervous system.

I'm a therapist, specifically a Chinese medicine therapist. Over the past few years, I've provided therapy called cycle breathing, bringing breath forward as a therapeutic tool, helping my patients on spiritual, emotional, and physical levels. It's like psychotherapy but not verbal. The use of continuous breathing alone clears emotional, physical, and spiritual poisons, making much needed internal space.

Holotropic breathing was invented by a Czech researcher in the 1970s after he had conducted extensive research with trauma using LSD in the 1960s, working with thousands of patients with notable success. Once LSD became illegal, he began looking for something similar that could offer comparable benefits. That's when he developed a method called holotropic breathing — a very intense, three-hour session. The more modern version that I use with my patients, called cycle breathing, is often closer to an hour long and gentler, yet still effective.

Trauma's connection to cycle breathing

Trauma starts when your body, your computer — your nervous system — is overwhelmed by too much information or input and doesn't know how to handle it. Trauma begins when your breath stops. You can see the opposite with babies, who never stop breathing. Babies' entire bodies expand and contract continuously, unlike adults, whose breath is often very shallow. Babies use their diaphragm fully; their entire organ system is vivid and activated purely by breathing. Trauma starts when you stop breathing causing your emotions to stop moving or freezing; everything inside of you becomes like a closed boiling pot.

Think of someone having an anxiety attack: their breath becomes rapid and shallow instead of deep and calming. Most techniques for anxiety involve deep breathing. Breath is the first step to keeping in motion, whether giving birth, experiencing orgasm, or balancing hormones as well as helping the immune system.

Trauma means you need to return to specific points and breathe into emotions and encourage your body to process events that occurred.

Right breathing

When the diaphragm is working, it helps you extract good hormones that balance your system, including your immune system. It's all a cycle. Breathing helps you stay in motion within this balanced thriving cycle.

When you are stuck in trauma, it means you need to come back to breath. This is what I do in my work, bringing the breath forward as a therapeutic tool that supports the human body on all levels: spiritual, emotional, and physical.

Breath will bring you back into your body.

Breathing sessions for therapeutic breath: Rebirthing

The treatments I do with my patients are 45 minutes to an hour of non-stop breathing, allowing emotions and physical pains to arise without giving the emotions the stage. Using continuous breath to heal. I instruct my clients to give full intention to breathing without stopping, holding space and ensuring the breathing is continuous the whole time — inhaling through the nose and exhaling through the mouth with a wide-open mouth. The idea is to exhale as many toxins as possible. The process is not meant to be rough or aggressive.

The concept is to allow emotions and sensations to move through without interruption. When emotions or insights arise, acknowledge them briefly and continue breathing, maintaining the flow.

In this kind of session, *things* come up. Emotions, memoires, events often arise. Sometimes physical pain surfaces. Breathe into them and continue the breath. The practice is to remind you that beneath your thoughts, emotions, and even pain, there's something very simple, very intact — a connection to deeper parts of yourself.

Breathing helps clean *things* out — from the organs, the skin, the muscles. It's very simple and very primal.

If the client breathes with a barely open mouth, it's very different than when they open their mouth wide and let all the air and emotion out, their body starts to process. After a few minutes, the body enters a trance. Emotions, memories, pain, cramps, or visions can arise. The key is overcome the natural urge to connect to the reaction, and to instead keep breathing. After the session ends is when to reflect on what came up — not during.

During the session, the client lies down,
closes their eyes, and breathes.

Sometimes I place hands on specific parts of the body — usually the chakras — to bring attention there. There is a simple way to diagnose which chakra is blocked. No need to say anything, just placing a hand can bring focus.

When something intense comes up, the breath rhythm changes — faster, stronger — until it releases. The release often ends in crying, screaming, or laughing and then settling. Breathing becomes whole and slow again. The body relaxes.

A person can experience one to 20 integrations in a single session.

Emotions can get stuck when we don't fully feel them, especially during trauma. Breathwork gives the body permission to feel, integrate, and release those stored emotions. It doesn't matter which emotion or when it happened. Through breathing, you can let it out. Integration often happens days later when the intellectual and emotional align.

At the end of a session, I play Tibetan bowls or my flute to help shift my patient into rest mode.

To integrate: cellular space and the spirit

What do I mean by integrate?

Integration relates to emotions and the internal systems. When emotions become stuck, they don't just remain somewhere abstract; they become trapped physically within your body — in your cells and tissues. These trapped emotions occupy spaces that ideally should remain open, spaces where our spirit naturally resides.

The spirit resides within the open spaces inside your body, particularly in hollow organs like the heart, liver, kidneys, spleen, and lungs. Emotions become trapped and fill these spaces, thus displacing the spirit and disrupting your sense of well-being.

When someone is continuously experiencing pain or negativity, they may forget what it feels like when things are internally good and peaceful.

Integration, therefore, refers to the process that occurs after a therapeutic session, where these emotional blockages are cleared, reopening the spaces so the spirit can comfortably reside there again.

Once the spirit can inhabit these open spaces, new ideas, inspirations, and insights naturally arise. Integration can sometimes take several days as the body readjusts to having this renewed openness.

Why is being calm so important?

Calmness allows one to clear and maintain these open spaces within the body. When you're calm, you create an environment where your spirit can effortlessly reside in softness, free from tension and struggle.

Letting go

There was a young woman with a lot of anger toward her mom, who was constantly intervening and criticizing. Her mom had some psychotic behaviors. As a young adult, this woman wanted to accept her mom, but she kept getting triggered. After four weekly Rebirthing sessions, she was able to accept her mother and, for the first time, set boundaries. She understood what she could and couldn't confront with her mom, and she stopped putting herself in triggering situations. During the sessions, she cried and screamed a lot; expressing what she was not able to in front of her mom.

The Rebirthing allowed her to release the stored anger and pain, no longer overrun by it.

Purging physically, mentally, emotionally, and spiritually

An important thing to understand is that the main function of our entire organ system is purification or detoxification. Its entire job is to purify the blood.

The lungs are the primary organ that help purify the blood in the most immediate way. When you take a big inhale and a big exhale, you are releasing a lot of toxins, including CO_2. When you are conscious about your breathing — especially in a moment when something hard or challenging is happening — it's essential to exhale as much as possible.

Like in the story I earlier shared with animals. When something brutal happens, they breathe very heavily.

So purging isn't only physical — it's mental, emotional, and spiritual too. If something very emotional is happening and you stop breathing, it likely evolves into trauma. But if you breathe, you support your system to digest it and release the toxins. You are then left with the realization of what's going on instead of freezing.

It's like a child who's very angry. A parent who sits down with them and says, "I see you're angry. Let's breathe together." This supports the child in being able to quickly calm down and become aware of what they're feeling — anger.

One client came to me for his first rebirthing session. He had a lot of trauma, especially related to his dad. His father had molested him, and although he had mentally accepted his father as a person and tried to move on, his emotions regarding his dad remained negative. After the session, he told me that during the breathwork, he revisited his own birth in a vision. He saw himself coming out of the womb, and in the vision, the first person who held him was his father. It was emotionally impactful because, for the first time in his 42 years, he saw his dad in a positive light — as a caring father, not the abuser.

The breathwork allowed him to have a somatic, emotional deep shift.

For example, I might say, "Oh yes, I'm feeling very angry," but in the breathwork, it doesn't matter why I'm angry. I go to the source and release it from there. In daily life, so many things happen that trigger us, like a fight with mom two days ago, or a conflict with a partner two weeks ago. It builds up. And breath clears it out.

Daily breath

The best way to breathe in daily life is inhaling through the nose and exhaling through the mouth. Nose breathing cools and cleans air, directing it to the lower abdomen, engaging the diaphragm, the largest muscle dividing chest and abdomen. Proper breathing involves the diaphragm expanding and contracting freely, facilitating nerve flow and calming the body.

Ideal posture for correct breathing

Posture significantly influences breathing. Aligning your spine allows your diaphragm to move freely. Sitting without back support for short periods strengthens spine muscles and encourages correct breathing posture. It's important that your feet remain grounded, signaling wholeness to the nervous system. Avoid crossing your legs excessively.

Emotionally and spiritually, correct breathing creates space within you. It allows emotions to move through without consuming you, fostering awareness rather than identifying with emotions. Breathing creates space for compassion and higher emotional states.

---

*Acknowledging emotions without becoming them
is central to emotional and spiritual health.*

Exercise to ground and feel calm in under a minute

This simple, brief exercise significantly will calm and center you, connecting deeply to your emotional and energetic bodies.

Let's practice a short breathing technique: take three breaths, hold the third inhale briefly, tap firmly on the sternum, and then exhale. This activates heart energy, signaling calmness and presence. Repeat three rounds for an immediate feeling of calm and grounding.

Do this three times, and at the end, I want you to notice how your breathing feels. We're going to do three rounds — three breaths, repeated three times.

And then coming back to normal breathing.

You likely feel more calm and more ease — and also more "alive" in an active present way.

You can do this short technique anytime you're feeling stressed or not inside your body.

In Chinese medicine, the heart is the emperor. The heart holds everything, and by giving a stamp of your awareness, that awareness goes into every cell of your body.

By tapping on the sternum, you're activating your heart. You're giving a strong vibration inside your chest while you are breathing. This sternum — this bone you have in your chest — can hold a lot of pressure. And by tapping strongly on it, you bring vibration inside your heart. You're saying, "Hey, wake up. Are you there? Are you okay?"

You can perform this technique anytime. It gives a lot of presence and calmness in the span of a minute.

Contraindications:

I wouldn't recommend this breathing exercise for someone with very low blood pressure, because it does bring the blood pressure down a bit. If you experience dizziness or feeling weak, refrain from this exercise.

My own healing breath story

Before my own series of rebirthing sessions, I believed that to achieve something, I had to give 200 percent of myself. I had huge expectations and ended up exhausted. During the first five sessions, I experienced intense pain in my body. I didn't understand why. Then I realized I was pushing too hard — not just in breathing but also in life. When I started breathing in my sessions with less effort and with more ease, I felt light, pleasure, even orgasmic sensations. I felt good with myself. I learned that I could give 70-80 percent with intention and still achieve my goals without overextending.

The result in my daily life? I now have more energy at the end of the day instead of being exhausted. I found a new way to approach achievement through breath.

Using breath in real time

After the burial of my dog, I lay on the hammock and started breathing. After five minutes, I cried. It helped me release. It took me out of the functional autopilot and into moving emotions through me.

I use breathwork, not always in formal sessions, but also while running — I practice staying focused on my breath.

During military training, before entering a warzone, where I was a logistics commander. One young soldier had a panic attack. Someone called me. I came, removed his gear, and walked him away. I didn't let him stop focusing on his breathing. For over an hour and a half, I kept repeating, "Keep breathing. Focus on your breath."

His mind was panicked, full of thoughts. I told him, "It's not time to think. Just breathe."

Afterward, we could talk. He said he didn't feel ready to fight but still wanted to contribute. He decided to join the logistics team and was incredibly helpful.

Breath helped him exit panic, connect to his truth, and make a clear decision. And without guilt or shame.

My weekly breathwork practice I recommend

Typically, I do an hour session once a week for myself; I block another hour after, free of any to-dos, so I don't feel rushed. Usually, my sessions are 45 minutes of breathing and at least 15 minutes of shavasana — a yogic form of active rest. That final relaxation is better than any drug — trust me.

Walking medicine: Diaphragm and psoas awareness

Something interesting about breathing — specifically, diaphragmatic breathing — is that the diaphragm is a huge muscle that separates the upper and lower parts of the body. It's the only organ directly connected to the heart. There's also an internal muscle connected to the diaphragm, called the psoas, which is one of the most important muscles in your body because it holds the main artery. In Hebrew, we call it "Avi," which translates to "the father of the artery."

If the psoas is relaxed, there's no tension on the artery. When you breathe properly and the diaphragm contracts and releases as it should, it stimulates the psoas to function at its highest potential. But when you sit with poor posture, you put pressure on the psoas, which can stagnate blood flow and create tension. So, it works both ways: proper breathing relaxes the psoas, and proper posture supports easier breathing.

If you're sitting poorly and try to breathe deeply, you'll often hit blockages. Interestingly, the one activity where this system works optimally and naturally is walking. When you walk, the diaphragm functions well, and the psoas, being a hip flexor, massages the diaphragm through the movement of your hips. It's a beautiful feedback system. The diaphragm is essentially the engine for your internal organs. When it moves well, the whole system benefits: blood flows better, digestion improves, and energy increases.

Prescription to walk

For people who don't do any physical activity and mostly sit all day, the minimum recommendation is three times per week for 30 minutes. And it doesn't have to be fast or intense — just consistent movement.

Walking is the most natural action you can do that preserves more energy than other exercise. Running, for example, consumes more energy, stresses the joints, and requires longer recovery. Walking offers a profound benefit with minimal downside.

There's one more thing I want to note, especially around exercise and breath. The most important part of breathing in exercise is the exhalation. Why? Because the pace of our resting breath is determined by the amount of CO_2 in our blood. Breathing is more about detoxification than it is about inhaling oxygen. Oxygen is easy for the body to access, but expelling toxins through the breath takes more effort.

When you exercise, you want to emphasize the exhale. That's where the real benefit is. When you exhale deeply, you support emotional and physical detoxification. It doesn't matter what kind of exercise you're doing — it's the exhalation that really matters.

In a natural state, everyone has access to enough oxygen. What differs is how much toxicity, physical and emotional, your body is carrying.

Your exhale is vital.

Final thoughts

Human potential is the feeling of goodness: feeling good with my body, good with my emotions, good in social encounters, and good with everything around me. It means using minimum energy to achieve the maximum result.

Thank you for your focus on this therapeutic tool, trusting it, and understanding that exploring our human potential brings more light into our lives and the lives of others. I'm grateful for the opportunity to contribute and share this powerful practice.

Key takeaways to implement

* In your daily life, and especially when experiencing hard emotions or challenging events, intentionally self-regulate with long exhalations (8+ seconds) breathing in through your nose and exhaling out through your mouth.
* Walk regularly, as medicine, for the diaphragm and nervous system. Minimum 3 times a week for 30 minutes. Focus on your exhale to release CO_2 and emotions.
* Use a guided breathwork session like holotropic or rebirthing to release stuck emotions and create internal space for your spirit.

About the author

Yotam Tamari is a man of peace and healing. Through his Chinese medicine studies, he built a bodywork practice using Tui Na. Tui Na is a traditional Chinese medicine (TCM) practice, specifically a form of therapeutic massage. It's based on the same principles as acupuncture, aiming to harmonize the body's Qi (energy flow) through manual manipulation.

Beyond his Tui Na practice he has become fascinated and passionate about the healing benefits of breath work to move and heal trauma that gets stuck in the body.

When he is not working, he is spending time with loved ones, celebrating life, and running with his dog.

To learn more and get in touch, email: yotamtamari@gmail.com

Psychedelic healing was one of the topics I specifically sought for this book. The paradigm shift from "drugs damage your brain" to "psychedelics can heal your brain" represents a truth I believe essential to share with those seeking deeper healing and neurological restoration.

Burton's work bridges traditional neurology with emerging psychedelic science for groundbreaking healing possibilities.

— *Book momma Chandra*

13

Brain Healing with Psychedelics

Burton J. Tabaac, MD, FAHA

From the sacred plant medicines utilized by ancient cultures to the latest neuroscience breakthroughs, psychedelics have long been associated with profoundly altered states of consciousness that are proposed to promote healing benefits. These powerful compounds are revealing tantalizing potential to revolutionize our understanding of the human brain, consciousness, and mental health disease states.

In this chapter, I will take you on a journey through the brief history, neuroscience, therapeutic applications, and societal implications of psychedelic therapeutics. I will explore with you how these extraordinary molecules are poised to reshape the landscape of neurological and psychiatric treatment, and how they may hold the key to unlocking human potential on a profound scale.

A brief history: Ancient roots and modern renaissance

The use of psychedelics dates back millennia, woven into the spiritual and medicinal practices of indigenous cultures worldwide. The Aztecs revered psilocybin-containing mushrooms, known as "teonanácatl" or "flesh of the gods," as conduits to the divine[1]. In the Amazon, ayahuasca, a brew containing the potent psychedelic DMT, has been used for centuries in sacred healing ceremonies.

The modern era of psychedelic research began in 1938, when Swiss chemist Albert Hofmann first synthesized lysergic acid diethylamide (LSD). Hofmann's accidental ingestion of LSD in 1943 sparked a wave of scientific interest in the compound's psychological effects. Throughout the '50s and '60s, researchers explored the therapeutic potential of LSD and other psychedelics, treating conditions ranging from alcoholism to end-of-life anxiety. Controversy mounted in the early '60s which saw the rise of recreational psychedelic use, fueled by countercultural figures like Harvard's Timothy Leary and his controversial exhortation to "turn on, tune in, drop out." As psychedelics became associated with the anti-establishment ethos of the era, political backlash led to their criminalization and the abrupt halt of most research.

In recent decades, a new generation of astute scientists have cautiously revived the study of psychedelics. Rigorous clinical trials, using modern protocols and safeguards, are demonstrating the therapeutic efficacy of these compounds for a range of mental health conditions. Universities like Johns Hopkins, Imperial College London, and the University of California, Berkeley have established dedicated psychedelic research centers, signaling a new chapter in the scientific understanding of these powerful substances. Quite dissimilar with the way in which these drugs were used in the '60s and '70s, there is now a more targeted approach for the way in which these medicines can be offered.

The neuroscience of psychedelics: Neuroplasticity and expanded consciousness

Psychedelics exert their profound effects by interacting with specific receptors in the brain, particularly serotonin receptors. The classic psychedelics, such as LSD, psilocybin, and DMT, activate the 5-HT2A serotonin receptor, triggering a cascade of neurochemical events that alter perception, cognition, and emotion. One of the most striking findings from modern neuroimaging studies is that psychedelics decrease activity in the brain's default mode network (DMN). The DMN is a collection of interconnected brain regions that is active when we are engaged in self-referential thought, mind-wandering, and rumination. Overactivity in the DMN has been linked to depression, anxiety, and other mental health disorders. By temporarily suppressing the DMN, psychedelics may allow the brain to break free from rigid, habitual patterns of thought and explore new avenues of neural connectivity.

Interestingly, psychedelics have been demonstrated to enhance neuroplasticity, the brain's ability to rewire itself and form new connections. This heightened plasticity may underlie the long-lasting therapeutic effects observed in many patients, as the brain forges new pathways that bypass entrenched patterns of negative thought and behavior. The interconnected areas of the DMN are very active in states of depression and anxiety, yet temporarily are inhibited when under the influence of psychedelics. A dedicated meditation practice also taps into and can inhibit the DMN, in which mindfulness allows for self-awareness and can promote personal growth.

Think of your mind as a snow-covered hill in which your thoughts are sleds. Over time, the grooves are dug deeper and deeper, making it difficult to escape the paths that are created. These paths, representative of our internal dialogue, then become ingrained. Psychedelics allow for a proverbial fresh mound of snow to be laid, which allows for new paths, thoughts, connections, and interpretations to be made. This may explain how psychedelics are effective at treating the ruminating thoughts consistent with addiction, anxiety, and depression.

The subjective psychedelic experience is crucially shaped by "set and setting" the user's mindset and the physical and social environment in which the medicine is taken. A supportive, guided therapeutic setting can channel the psychedelic experience toward personal insight, emotional catharsis, and positive transformation. Conversely, uncontrolled or adverse settings can lead to distressing or unpredictable outcomes, underscoring the importance of careful preparation and supervision in both research and clinical contexts.

Psychedelics and mental health: Treating the pathological mind

The most robust evidence for the therapeutic potential of psychedelics comes from studies on depression, anxiety, PTSD, and addiction. Psilocybin, in particular, has shown impressive results in treating these conditions, often with just one or two guided sessions. In a landmark 2016 study, a single dose of psilocybin produced rapid and sustained reductions in depression symptoms in patients with treatment-resistant depression. Remarkably, 67 percent of participants showed clinically significant improvements, and 58 percent achieved complete remission at 5 weeks post-treatment[2]. Follow-up studies have found that these benefits can endure for months or even years, suggesting that psilocybin may induce lasting changes in brain function and connectivity, which could account for the enduring therapeutic effects observed[3].

Similar results have been observed for anxiety, particularly in patients with life-threatening illnesses. A 2016 randomized controlled trial found that a single dose of psilocybin, combined with psychotherapy, led to significant reductions in anxiety and depression in patients with advanced-stage cancer. These effects were sustained for at least six months, and participants reported increased quality of life, acceptance, and spiritual wellbeing[4].

PTSD, a notoriously difficult condition to treat, has revealed remarkable promise in early psychedelic trials. MDMA, sometimes considered a psychedelic due to its empathogenic and mildly hallucinogenic effects, has been designated a "breakthrough therapy" by the FDA for PTSD treatment. In Phase 2 clinical trials, MDMA-assisted psychotherapy led to significant reductions in PTSD symptoms, with 68 percent of participants no longer meeting diagnostic criteria for PTSD at 12-month follow-up[5].

Addiction has the profound propensity to yield to psychedelic interventions. Psilocybin has shown efficacy in treating tobacco, alcohol, and cocaine addiction, while ibogaine, a psychedelic derived from the African iboga plant, has been used to interrupt opioid addiction. These substances seem to work by disrupting compulsive drug-seeking behavior, reducing cravings, and promoting insight and motivation for change[6-9].

Psychedelics and neurological diseases: Regenerating the brain

Beyond mental health, psychedelics are underscoring intriguing potential in the treatment of neurological conditions such as stroke, traumatic brain injury, and neurodegenerative diseases like dementia. Stroke and traumatic brain injury often result in chronic neurological deficits due to limited spontaneous recovery and the brain's diminished capacity for repair. By enhancing neuroplasticity, psychedelics may help the brain rewire itself and regain lost function. Animal studies have shown that psychedelics can stimulate the growth of new neurons, increase synaptic connections, and promote the formation of new neural networks[10,11]. While human research in this area is still nascent, case reports and small studies suggest that psychedelics may indeed aid recovery from brain injury[12].

In the realm of neurodegenerative diseases, psychedelics are being explored as potential treatments for conditions like Alzheimer's and Parkinson's disease. These disorders are characterized by the progressive loss of neurons and synaptic connections, leading to cognitive decline, memory loss, and motor impairment. By stimulating neurogenesis and synaptogenesis, psychedelics may help slow or even reverse the course of neurodegeneration. Ayahuasca, in particular, has shown promise in this regard. The brew contains harmine, a compound that has been shown to stimulate the formation of new neurons and protect against oxidative stress and inflammation, key factors in neurodegenerative processes. Preclinical studies have found that harmine can improve cognitive function and reduce amyloid plaques, a hallmark of Alzheimer's disease[13].

In a highly compelling study, Dr. Gül Dölen, MD, PhD and her team uncovered a shared mechanism across psychedelic drugs that could explain their similar subjective effects and therapeutic benefits. By demonstrating that psychedelics can reopen the critical period for social reward learning in adult mice, a window of heightened neuroplasticity typically confined to early development, the researchers provide a unifying framework for understanding how these substances influence the brain. Intriguingly, the duration of this reopened critical period in mice correlates with the reported timeline of acute subjective effects in humans. These findings not only shed light on the fundamental neurobiology of psychedelics but also have important implications for their clinical application and the development of novel therapies[14].

While much more research is needed to fully understand the potential of psychedelics in neurological disorders, these early findings suggest a promising new avenue for treatment and neuroprotection. Some have posited that psychedelics address the underlying problem leading to mental health woes while the current accepted standard of care prescribed simply addresses symptoms.

From single dose to lasting transformation

One of the most remarkable aspects of psychedelic therapy is the potential for long-lasting, even transformative effects from just one or a few doses. This stands in stark contrast to traditional psychiatric medications, which often require daily administration and may lose efficacy over time. The mechanisms underlying this long-term benefit are not fully understood, but likely involve a combination of neurobiological and psychological factors. On the neurobiological level, psychedelics may induce lasting changes in brain connectivity and function, "resetting" neural circuits and allowing for the emergence of new patterns of thought and behavior. The enhanced neuroplasticity triggered by psychedelics may enable the brain to "learn" and internalize therapeutic insights and coping strategies.

On the psychological level, the profound, often mystical-type experiences occasioned by psychedelics can lead to enduring shifts in perspective, self-understanding, and worldview. Many patients report a renewed sense of meaning, purpose, and interconnectedness following psychedelic therapy. These existential insights may serve as a catalyst for long-term behavioral change and emotional healing. The long-lasting nature of psychedelic therapy also has important implications for accessibility and cost-effectiveness. If a single dose can produce enduring benefits, psychedelic treatments could potentially reach a much larger population than traditional pharmacotherapy or psychotherapy, which require ongoing sessions and resources.

Psychedelic integration is a crucial aspect of optimizing the transformative potential that arises from psychedelic experiences. After encountering the profound depths of altered consciousness induced by substances like psilocybin, LSD, or ayahuasca, it is essential to integrate the insights, epiphanies, and emotional breakthroughs into one's daily life.

Journaling allows individuals to capture and reflect upon the rich tapestry of their psychedelic experiences, facilitating a deeper understanding of the symbolic, emotional, and spiritual insights revealed. Mindfulness practices like meditation can help ground and embody the expansive states of awareness encountered during the psychedelic journey. Additionally, participating in integration circles or seeking the guidance of experienced psychedelic facilitators can provide a supportive framework for processing and contextualizing these profound experiences, promoting lasting personal growth and transformation.

Collective consciousness and impact at scale

Beyond their clinical applications, psychedelics are gaining attention for their potential to promote societal and cultural transformation. Some researchers and thinkers propose that widespread responsible use of psychedelics could lead to a collective waking up— a shift toward greater empathy, ecological awareness, and global consciousness.

The idea is that by inducing profound experiences of unity, inter-connectedness, and self-transcendence, psychedelics can help dissolve the boundaries of the ego and foster a sense of oneness with others and the natural world. This expanded perspective could, in theory, translate into more compassionate, cooperative, and sustainable behaviors on a societal level. While this vision remains speculative, there is some evidence that psychedelic experiences can indeed promote prosocial attitudes and behaviors.

Studies have found that psychedelic use is associated with increased openness, empathy, and concern for others, as well as reduced authoritarianism and prejudice[15,16]. Lifetime psychedelic use has also been associated with increased nature relatedness, which in turn predicted pro-environmental behavior; suggesting that psychedelic experiences can lead to a heightened sense of connection with nature and a greater concern for the environment[17].

It is crucial to note that the idea of psychedelics as a panacea for societal ills is overly simplistic and risks overlooking the complex social, political, and economic factors that shape our world. Psychedelics are not a magic bullet, and their beneficial effects are not guaranteed. Much depends on the context, intention, and integration of the psychedelic experience. Nevertheless, the notion of psychedelics as catalysts for positive social change is a compelling one and deserves further exploration and discussion. As research continues to illuminate the transformative potential of these substances, it is important to consider their implications not just for individual health, but for the collective wellbeing of our species and planet.

The evolving legal landscape

As scientific evidence for the therapeutic benefits of psychedelics mounts, the legal landscape is beginning to shift. In recent years, several jurisdictions have taken steps to recognize psychedelics as medicines and to reduce barriers to research and treatment. In 2019, the city of Denver became the first in the United States to decriminalize psilocybin mushrooms, followed by Oakland and Santa Cruz, California, which decriminalized all entheogenic plants and fungi. In 2020, the state of Oregon made history by legalizing psilocybin for therapeutic use, establishing a regulatory framework for psilocybin-assisted therapy.

Other countries are also moving toward more permissive policies. In 2019, Israel became the first country to approve compassionate use of MDMA-assisted psychotherapy for PTSD. In 2020, Canada granted exemptions to several patients with terminal illnesses to undergo psilocybin therapy, paving the way for broader access. Since July 2023, psychiatrists can be authorized to prescribe MDMA and psilocybin for use in psychedelic assisted psychotherapy to treat PTSD and treatment-resistant depression respectively.

These legal developments reflect a growing recognition of psychedelics as legitimate medical tools, and a shift away from the punitive drug policies of the past. However, progress remains slow, and psychedelics are still classified as Schedule I substances under U.S. federal law and international drug control conventions. Ongoing advocacy and education efforts aim to change this, by highlighting the scientific evidence, challenging stigma and misconceptions, and pushing for sensible, evidence-based policies. Organizations like the Multidisciplinary Association for Psychedelic Studies (MAPS), the Beckley Foundation, and the Usona Institute are working to advance psychedelic research and promote legal reforms.

As the legal landscape continues to evolve, it is crucial to prioritize safety, ethics, and equitable access in the development of psychedelic therapies. This includes establishing rigorous training and certification standards for therapists, ensuring informed consent and patient safeguards, and working to make treatments affordable and available to all who could benefit.

Final thoughts

The resurgence of psychedelic science is one of the most exciting and promising developments in the fields of neuroscience and mental health. From their ancient shamanic roots to the cutting edge of modern medicine, psychedelics are revealing new frontiers in our understanding of consciousness, the brain, and human potential. As research continues to unfold, it is becoming clear that psychedelics are not just tools for treating illness, but for fostering wellness, growth, and transformation. By enhancing neuroplasticity, facilitating insight and emotional processing, and promoting long-term changes in perspective and behavior, psychedelics may offer a paradigm shift in how we approach mental health and personal development.

The use of psychedelics raises important questions and challenges. How do we ensure safe, ethical, and equitable access to these powerful substances? How do we integrate psychedelic experiences into our lives and society in a way that maximizes their benefits and minimizes their risks? How do we harness the transformative potential of psychedelics while respecting the complexities of the human mind and the diversity of cultural contexts?

These are questions that will require ongoing dialogue, research, and reflection as the psychedelic renaissance unfolds. As we navigate this new and exciting territory, it is essential to approach psychedelics with humility, curiosity, and a commitment to science, compassion, and the expansion of human possibility. The future of psychedelic medicine is bright, and its implications are vast. With wisdom and care, we may be on the cusp of a new era in our understanding and cultivation of the mind, with profound consequences for individuals, society, and the world at large.

Notes

[1] Carod-Artal, F. J. (2015). Hallucinogenic drugs in pre-Columbian Mesoamerican cultures. *Neurología* (English Edition), 30(1), 42–49.

[2] Carhart-Harris, R. L., Bolstridge, M., Rucker, J., Day, C. M., Erritzoe, D., Kaelen, M., Bloomfield, M., Rickard, J. A., Forbes, B., Feilding, A., Taylor, D., Pilling, S., Curran, V. H., & Nutt, D. J. (2016). Psilocybin with psychological support for treatment-resistant depression: An open-label feasibility study. *The Lancet Psychiatry*, 3(7), 619–627.

[3] Carhart-Harris, R. L., Bolstridge, M., Day, C. M. J., Rucker, J., Watts, R., Erritzoe, D. E., Kaelen, M., Giribaldi, B., Bloomfield, M., Pilling, S., Rickard, J. A., Forbes, B., Feilding, A., Taylor, D., Curran, H. V., & Nutt, D. J. (2018). Psilocybin with psychological support for treatment-resistant depression: Six-month follow-up. *Psychopharmacology* (Berl), 235(2), 399–408. https://doi.org/10.1007/s00213-017-4771-x

[4] Griffiths, R. R., Johnson, M. W., Carducci, M. A., Umbricht, A., Richards, W. A., Richards, B. D., Cosimano, M. P., & Klinedinst, M. A. (2016). Psilocybin produces substantial and sustained decreases in depression and anxiety in patients with life-threatening cancer: A randomized double-blind trial. *Journal of Psychopharmacology*, 30(12), 1181–1197.

[5] Mithoefer, M. C., Mithoefer, A. T., Feduccia, A. A., Jerome, L., Wagner, M., Wymer, J., Holland, J., Hamilton, S., Yazar-Klosinski, B., Emerson, A., & Doblin, R. (2018). 3,4-Methylenedioxymethamphetamine (MDMA)-assisted psychotherapy for post-traumatic stress disorder in military veterans, firefighters, and police officers: A randomized, double-blind, dose-response, phase 2 clinical trial. *The Lancet Psychiatry*, 5(6), 486–497.

[6] Johnson, M. W., Garcia-Romeu, A., Cosimano, M. P., & Griffiths, R. R. (2014). Pilot study of the 5-HT2AR agonist psilocybin in the treatment of tobacco addiction. *Journal of Psychopharmacology*, 28(11), 983–992.

[7] Bogenschutz, M. P., Forcehimes, A. A., Pommy, J. A., Wilcox, C. E., Barbosa, P., & Strassman, R. J. (2015). Psilocybin-assisted treatment for

alcohol dependence: A proof-of-concept study. *Journal of Psychopharmacology*, 29(3), 289–299.

[8] Johnson, M. W., Garcia-Romeu, A., & Griffiths, R. R. (2017). Long-term follow-up of psilocybin-facilitated smoking cessation. *The American Journal of Drug and Alcohol Abuse*, 43(1), 55–60.

[9] Brown, T. K., & Alper, K. (2018). Treatment of opioid use disorder with ibogaine: Detoxification and drug use outcomes. *The American Journal of Drug and Alcohol Abuse*, 44(1), 24–36.

[10] Ly, C., Soltanzadeh Zarandi, S., Sood, A., Paddy, M. R., Duim, W. C., Dennis, M. Y., McAllister, A. K., Ori-McKenney, K. M., Gray, J. A., & Olson, D. E. (2018). Psychedelics promote structural and functional neural plasticity. *Cell Reports*, 23(11), 3170–3182.

[11] Shao, L. X., Liao, C., Gregg, I., Davoudian, P. A., Savalia, N. K., Delagarza, K., & Kwan, A. C. (2021). Psilocybin induces rapid and persistent growth of dendritic spines in frontal cortex in vivo. *Neuron*, 109(16), 2535–2544.e4.

[12] Cherian, K. N., Keynan, J. N., Anker, L., et al. (2024). Magnesium—ibogaine therapy in veterans with traumatic brain injuries. *Nature Medicine*, 30, 373–381.

[13] Zheng, X., Zhang, X., Kang, A., Ran, C., Wang, G., & Hao, H. (2015). Thinking outside the brain for cognitive improvement: Is peripheral immunomodulation on the way? *Neuropharmacology*, 96(Pt A), 94–104.

[14] Nardou, R., Sawyer, E., Song, Y. J., et al. (2023). Psychedelics reopen the social reward learning critical period. *Nature*, 618, 790–798.

[15] Nour, M. M., Evans, L., & Carhart-Harris, R. L. (2017). Psychedelics, personality and political perspectives. *Journal of Psychoactive Drugs*, 49(3), 182–191.

[16] Forstmann, M., Yudkin, D. A., Prosser, A. M., Heller, S. M., & Crockett, M. J. (2020). Transformative experience and social connectedness mediate the mood-enhancing effects of psychedelic use in naturalistic settings. *Proceedings of the National Academy of Sciences*, 117(5), 2338–2346.

[17] Forstmann, M., & Sagioglou, C. (2017). Lifetime experience with (classic) psychedelics predicts pro-environmental behavior through an increase in nature relatedness. *Journal of Psychopharmacology, 31*(8), 975–988.

Key takeaways to implement

* Educate yourself thoroughly on the potential benefits and risks of psychedelic-assisted therapies by consulting reputable scientific sources and expert opinions. As research rapidly advances in this field, stay informed about the latest findings unveiling the therapeutic applications of psychedelics for mental health conditions and neurological disorders.

* Advocate for evidence-based policies and increased access to psychedelic therapies. As legal reforms progress, amplify your voice through organizations promoting research, education, and sensible regulation, such as MAPS or the Beckley Foundation. Engage locally by joining psychedelic societies, integration circles, and advocating before state legislatures to shape the future of these promising treatments.

* Contemplate the profound insights, empathy, and interconnectedness fostered by psychedelic experiences—reflecting on how they could catalyze personal growth and positive societal transformation. Engage in thoughtful discourse around their transformative potential, while grounding discussions in scientific evidence and responsible use.

About the author

Burton J. Tabaac, MD, FAHA is an Associate Professor of Neurology at The University of Nevada, Reno School of Medicine, dedicated to the cutting-edge treatment and prevention of neurological diseases. He serves as the Section Chief of Neurology and Medical Director of Stroke affiliated with Carson Tahoe Health. Dr. Tabaac is a graduate of the fellowship program in cerebrovascular neurology at The Johns Hopkins University Hospital in Baltimore, MD (2019). After graduating from AUC School of Medicine, where he earned his MD (2014), Tabaac completed a neurology residency at Rutgers Robert Wood Johnson in New Bruns-wick, NJ. There, he was humbled to have been selected as a three-time recipient of The Arnold P. Gold Foundation's Humanism and Excellence in Teaching Award (2016, 2017, and 2018). Tabaac has been honored by being inducted into the Alpha Omega Alpha Honor Medical Society. In 2021 he was awarded the prestigious accolade of fellowship affiliation with the American Heart Association.

Tabaac's research interests in the psychedelics space are focused on the potential for healing traumatic brain injury and promoting rehabilita-tion in stroke patients. Tabaac served as a TEDx speaker in 2022 at UCLA, presenting a talk entitled, "Mental Health Meets Psychedelics." As of 2023, Tabaac has been welcomed as a Special Advisor to the Board for The McKenna Academy of Natural Philosophy. In 2024 he was appointed as a Member of the Psychedelic Medicines Working Group for Nevada State to provide expertise and testimony relating to the therapeutic use of entheogens, with presentations to the 83rd Session of the Nevada Legislature. As of 2025 he is working as a research clinician on the PHATHOM project under the guidance of Gül Dölen of UC Berkeley, pairing psilocybin and enriched environments to promote motor recov-ery after stroke.

YouTube - "Mental Health Meets Psychedelics |
Burton Tabaac | TEDxUCLA"
https://www.youtube.com/watch?v=yk-vcGyXaCA

Greg's Radiance Ketamine Clinic in Reno stands among the nation's finest. His story of discovering ketamine's potential for depression treatment marks a significant moment in mental health innovation. His work centers on helping people reclaim their lives from debilitating conditions.

His compassionate approach combines medical expertise with a genuine desire to alleviate suffering through this promising treatment option.

— Book momma Chandra

14

Ketamine for Mental Health

Greg Jones, CRNA, MS, BSN

I'm still shocked that I'm even in the field of psychedelic medicine. Growing up a devout Mormon in a small town in Idaho, psyche-delics were the farthest thing from my mind. I was a proud graduate of the Drug Abuse Resistance Education (D.A.R.E.) pro-gram, after all! I had been convinced that all psychedelic medicines would fry my brain like an egg.

So, when did that change? Well, one day while giving anesthesia at the University of California San Francisco (UCSF), one of my patients asked me if I would give him some ketamine while he was asleep. Sur-prised by this, I asked the gentleman the purpose of his unique request. He said that he was a psychiatrist, and had suffered from major depres-sion his entire life. He had read several studies describing ketamine's impressive antidepressant effects and wanted to see if it would work for him. After some contemplation, I obliged and was excited to talk with him when he woke up.

To my delight, he said that he felt remarkably better. That night, I went home and began researching ketamine's effect on depression and other mental health conditions. This ignited a passion within me and ul-timately led to my opening of Radiance Ketamine Clinic in Reno, Nevada and VividLife Ketamine Clinic in Concord, California.

Ketamine's radical change

All of my patients struggle with their mental health. They either have major depressive disorder (MDD), post-traumatic stress disorder (PTSD), general anxiety disorder (GAD), obsessive-compulsive disorder (OCD), or suicidal ideations (SI). Most have a combination of these conditions. They're hurting and just want to feel better. Although they're hopeful that ketamine will help them, they're also skeptical. They've tried numerous treatments in the past and nothing has worked. I truly believe that the reason the treatments haven't worked isn't because there's an issue with the patient; it's because there's an issue with the treatments. The patients haven't failed the treatments; the treatments have failed the patients.

Gratefully, many of my patients respond positively to their ketamine treatments. A recent analysis of my patients' response to ketamine revealed the following:

- 78.26 percent experience at least a 10 percent improvement in their depressive symptoms.

- Of those that responded positively, their PHQ-9 score (a scale that measures depressive symptoms) dropped by an average of 8.42 points.

- This means that their depression dropped by an average of two categories (e.g., from severe to moderate depression or moderate to minimal/no depression).

Such changes can have a drastic improvement on one's quality of life. They're frequently filled with positivity, relief and hope. Many make comments such as, "I feel like my old self again" or "ketamine saved my life."

The power of ketamine

From my experience, ketamine is a life-changing and life-saving medicine. I still remember the shock that I felt while treating one of my very first patients. She had struggled with severe depression since childhood and had tried almost every antidepressant on the market. She then developed PTSD after witnessing her partner's death. The paramedics performed CPR on him for over an hour, trying to bring him back to life. She was racked with vivid nightmares and flashbacks, causing her depression to plummet even further. These dark feelings triggered suicidal thoughts. She didn't know if she could hold on much longer. We started treatment and after a few sessions, she said to me, "I think it's gone." I asked her what she was referring to and she said, "My PTSD." I was taken aback. I had read studies about ketamine's potent effects but to see them in action like that nearly took my breath away. She and I cried together out of true gratitude.

I went into medicine because I wanted to make a difference, a real difference in the world and in my patients' lives. I was beginning to realize that this dream was finally coming to fruition. I was truly humbled to see this radical change and to be part of my patient's healing journey.

How ketamine works

Research has revealed that ketamine works in a few different ways.

The first is through the neurophysiological changes that ketamine causes within the brain itself. Although the extent of ketamine's effect is still not fully understood, scientists believe that ketamine interacts with many different pathways within our brain. One of the predominant ways is by blocking the NMDA (N-methyl-D-aspartate) receptor.[6,7,21] I won't bore you with the intricate details of this complex neuronal unit but what it ultimately does is it increases the release of a substance called **glutamate**.[4,6,9,13] Glutamate is the most abundant stimulatory chemical in the brain.[1,7] A very simplistic description of it would be to compare it to fertilizer. When it is released, it activates neurons.[1] As a result, this can stimulate them to grow, increase their activity and help them connect with other neurons.[4,6,7] These changes can be so drastic that they can even be visualized on various medical scans of the brain.[4,6,9,16,17,21]

You may have heard the term neuroplasticity before. It's become a buzzword over the last several years. It is our brain's ability to adapt and change to its environment. It allows us to respond to situations that we encounter throughout our lives.[14] It is believed that when we are young, our minds are very plastic and moldable, but over time, and in certain conditions like depression, this moldability decreases.[4,15] Ketamine has been shown to increase a substance in our brains called **Brain-Derived Neurotrophic Factor** (BDNF), which in turn, increases neuroplasticity.[4,7,9,20]

As you can imagine, increasing the firing capability of our neurons and their ability to respond to daily life can have a substantial impact on our mood. These are just two of the over 10 different ways that scientists believe that ketamine helps improve brain function, and therefore, one's mental health.[7,8,9,10,12,17,20] Studies continue to unveil in more detail how exactly ketamine exerts its impressive effects on the brain.

Another important way that ketamine works is that it can produce an **extraordinary state of consciousness**. We'll go over what this may feel like in more detail later on but being able to process things with your "ketamine mind" is another important way that ketamine can improve mental health.

It's important to note, however, that while this altered state can provide many healing benefits, it may not be required for ketamine to exert its positive effects on mental health. Studies vary on whether or not this state is actually necessary.[3,9,20] Based on my clinical experience, I believe that this extraordinary state can and does provide many healing benefits. However, I've also seen patients' mental health improve without entering into this state at all. I mention this because many people correlate ketamine's beneficial effects solely on the altered state, which I don't believe to be true.

Types of ketamine

There are currently two forms of ketamine that can be given in the United States for mental health; racemic ketamine and esketamine.

The oldest form of ketamine, **racemic ketamine**, has been around since the 1960s.[7] It's been used as an anesthetic agent for both humans and animals for decades.[8] Its ability to improve depression was first discovered in the 1990s.[8] Doctors have been providing this form of ketamine for mental health since the late 2000s.[12] It's usually administered as an IV infusion, an injection or taken orally. This form of ketamine is not usually covered by insurance plans to treat mental health conditions at this time.

Racemic ketamine is made up of two halves called S-ketamine and R-ketamine.[7] They're like your hands. They look the same but they aren't exactly. There are some differences between the two halves but, in general, they are very similar to each other.

The second form of ketamine is S-ketamine alone. This medication goes by the brand name **Spravato** or the generic name **esketamine**.[18] Spravato was FDA-approved in 2019 for major depressive disorder (MDD) that has not responded to two or more oral antidepressants.[2,5] In 2020, the FDA also approved Spravato for those with MDD that are also acutely suicidal.[11] This form of ketamine is covered by almost all insurance plans, as long as you meet their qualifying criteria.

The ketamine experience

Believe me when I say that it's extremely difficult to describe how ketamine makes you feel. The reason is because every person is different and every ketamine session is unique. If you end up trying ketamine one day, you'll understand what I mean when you try to explain your experience to others.

The best way that I can think of to describe it is to compare it to having a daydream. When you open your eyes, you're in your treatment room. When you close your eyes, you're in a transient dream-like state.

The first thing that you'll likely feel when it starts to kick in is a deep sense of relaxation. Then you may notice more physical sensations, like seeing geometric shapes, a slight numbness around your mouth, ringing in your ears or heaviness in your arms and legs because you're just so relaxed. Then your mind usually becomes more active. This can be a mixture of things, such as replaying life experiences, visualizing your aspirations, or releasing suppressed emotions. It will likely be a mixture of these.

Sometimes your experiences will be random and won't seem to follow any kind of flow. Other times they'll be very direct and have a specific theme. Some sessions are more intense while others are more light and floaty. I keep saying this but every treatment will be different. That's part of the beauty of them. Learning to let go of control and just "going with the flow" is one of the great lessons that I believe ketamine teaches its receptive students.

As a medical provider, it is a true privilege to offer this amazing treatment to my patients. To watch them heal right in front of my eyes is the most divine thing that I can think of. Granted, not every ketamine session is life-altering but being able to sit with patients when deep, meaningful sessions occur makes me passionate about what I do every day.

Bad experiences

I don't believe that there are "bad trips." I believe that there are challenging experiences that bring up powerful emotions. These are frequently the most therapeutic sessions, however, because of their proximity to the core of what you're trying to address. Just as if you were mining for diamonds, initially the diamond may be filthy and covered in dirt. Once you clean it off though, you're left with this beautiful treasure.

That's also why it's so vital that you trust the people that are providing your treatments. Your trust in them will let your mind relax and allow it to go to difficult places. That's where the really good stuff is.

Ketamine's legal status

Ketamine is currently the only legal psychedelic medicine available in most areas of the country as a treatment for mental health. Hopefully this will change in the future, but that is where we stand as of early 2025. Ketamine must be prescribed by a medical provider.

Maximizing your ketamine sessions

There are a number of things that you can do to increase the efficacy of your treatments. These recommendations apply not only to ketamine treatments but to any psychedelic treatment, as they become legally accessible in the future.

1. **"Set and Setting."** This is a term that was popularized by Timothy Leary regarding psychedelic use.

   Set refers to the mindset you have when taking any mind-altering substance. As I mentioned previously, your frame of mind when you receive ketamine can greatly affect your treatment. For that reason, I recommend that you come to your sessions feeling calm and grounded. I understand that this is not always possible but taking a moment or two to clear your mind before starting your treatment can greatly influence your experience.

   Setting refers to the physical setting in which you receive the medication. Examples of this include the room that you are in, the team providing your treatment, whether or not you're on your phone, the music that you listen to, and who's in the room with you. All of these can affect your experience. Prepare your setting so that it's the most conducive to healing it can be. I recommend patients *not* bring a friend or loved one with them into their treatment room, even though it is commonly desired to do so. The reason is because patients who do, tend to find the accompanying person to be a distraction to their inner healing journey.

2. **Your focus.** Selecting an intention of what you'd like to focus on during your treatment can greatly influence your session as well. Common intentions include forgiving oneself, letting go of control, and showing more compassion to one's partner. I find that it's best to set your intention at least a few days prior to your ketamine treatment; the earlier the better. That way it gives you time to really reflect on your selected intention. By doing so, you're planting the seed in your mind. When you come in for your treatment, however, I recommend opening up your mind and seeing where it wants to take you. Don't force yourself to think about your intention. You're more likely to think about it because you've planted the seed but you may very well not think about it. You may think about it in three sessions or in five sessions and that's ok. It's all part of the healing process and letting go of control.

3. **Hide your phone.** We are on our phones all day. Set this time aside for you and your mental health. This treatment is all about you. You don't want to be distracted for it.

4. **Bathroom break.** Ketamine usually makes you need to urinate, so stop by the bathroom before things get started.

5. **Your tunes.** The type of music that you choose to listen to while on ketamine will have a powerful impact on your session. You'll find that the music really guides your thoughts and shapes your experience. So much so that when the song changes, your thoughts usually do as well.

   Here are a few ideas regarding your ketamine music:

   a. I generally recommend listening to music without lyrics or in a language that you don't understand. The reason is because people tend to hyperfocus on the words in the songs rather than on the experience itself.

   b. Listening to music that you're not familiar with stimulates your mind to explore new areas, rather than just jamming out to your favorite tunes.

   c. Playlists that have a mixture of lighter and more intense music seem to be the most therapeutic. Intense music can elicit stronger thoughts and emotions, while lighter music can facilitate their release.

   d. You can make your own playlists or search for ketamine playlists that others have created and made available on music platforms.

   e. If you do use a music platform, having a premium account will prevent you from getting an advertisement in the middle of your session.

   f. Preselecting a few playlists allows you to move between them throughout your sessions as you see fit.

   g. Using good quality, noise-cancelling headphones can really make a difference as well.

6. **Inward or outward.** Covering your eyes or keeping them closed will usually intensify your session. Most patients find that keeping their eyes open causes them to concentrate on external objects, like a loved one in the room. Keeping them closed, allows them to direct their focus inward, onto themselves. Depending on what you want to focus on that day, you may consider keeping your eyes open or leaving them closed.

7. **Objects.** Bringing something that you want to focus on can be helpful, such as a photo or keepsake from a loved one. You may also want to bring a grounding object, such as a favorite blanket or a stuffed animal.

8. **Journaling.** Taking notes of the things that came up during your sessions can be invaluable. Sometimes you'll think about very deep, emotional topics that carry a lot of meaning. Other times

you'll think about random stuff that doesn't seem to make a whole lot of sense. Either way, taking notes about each session and reflecting on those notes afterward frequently brings them to light and reveals their hidden meaning.

9. **Talk therapy.** I strongly encourage combining ketamine with psychotherapy. Unlike many antidepressants that tend to numb your feelings and shove issues down deeper, ketamine tends to bring things up and puts them in your face. Having a trained therapist that you can discuss these topics with can be extremely beneficial.

10. **Integration.** A key part of treatment is not just getting the ketamine treatment itself but implementing the insights that you received during your treatments into your life. This is called integration. Let's say that you have a very therapeutic session but do nothing with it. It will just remain this really great ketamine session but will have little to no impact on your actual life. People hear about how powerful ketamine can be, and it's absolutely true. The real power, however, usually comes from ketamine revealing the roadblocks in your life and *you* taking the necessary steps to remove them. It's hard work but that's what really brings about the positive changes in your life. Changes that you can actually feel.

Adverse effects

Virtually all of my prospective patients are worried about ketamine's potential side effects, and rightfully so. They've tried antidepressants and usually stopped them because of these effects, particularly emotional numbing, weight gain, and sexual dysfunction.

Gratefully, I've never had any patients experience a significant adverse reaction to ketamine. Almost all negative side effects occur during the ketamine session itself and wear off soon after the treatment is done. These include symptoms such as nausea, headache, feeling drunk, elevated blood pressure, dizziness, sedation and drowsiness. These do not usually occur every session and are generally well-tolerated. They also tend to decrease in intensity the more treatments that you receive.

There is also the potential for more significant side effects, such as inflammation of the bladder, ulcers in the bladder, liver impairment, vascular ruptures and an allergic reaction. Again, I've never seen these happen, since they usually occur in a non-medical setting and when very large doses of ketamine are consumed regularly. Although uncommon, these side effects can occur.

In addition, you will likely become dissociated and lose touch with reality while on ketamine. For this reason, and the potential side effects listed above, it's vital that ketamine be administered in a safe, medical setting. Consuming ketamine on your own, even if it's prescribed by a doctor, may put you in a potentially vulnerable and unsafe situation; which is not something that I recommend.

Real-life ketamine results

I'm frequently asked what are the usual results that I see from ketamine treatments. Just as all of my patients are unique, so are their individual results. Having said that, I've definitely seen trends in the approximate 20,000 ketamine and Spravato treatments that I have provided and supervised over the years.

1. **Mind chatter.** Most of us have a voice in our heads that seems to always be talking. Within a few treatments, most patients begin commenting on how that voice has changed. It usually becomes softer, gentler, and sometimes stops all together.

2. **The ketamine split-second.** Impulsivity is something that many of my patients struggle with. They tend to respond to situations based on their emotions at the time, often regretting their actions later. Although ketamine doesn't usually completely eliminate this, it can provide a split-second pause. This allows the patient to make more logical decisions, rather than just relying on their

emotions to make decisions for them. Ketamine can increase their cognitive-emotional flexibility.

3. **Rediscovery of hobbies.** Those suffering from depression have witnessed first-hand its ability to drain the satisfaction out of their hobbies. Gratefully, ketamine can help them reclaim that passion. So much of the art in my clinics was given to me by my patients. They are so grateful that ketamine has reawakened their passion for art. This alone can have dramatic effects on one's appetite for life.

4. **Reframing past experiences.** If you're like most people, you've probably experienced some painful events in your life. An important way to reduce the pain that these events can carry is to reframe them; removing their emotional punch. It's difficult to do that, however, because any time you get close to them, the pain they emanate pushes you away. Ketamine can provide a unique ability to unwrap these experiences without being triggered. It can change the angle from which you see them. It's almost like ketamine allows you to see them from a third-person perspective. Like an outsider looking in, rather than confronting them head on. This adjustment in perspective may allow you to change how you view these events and, therefore, the impact that they have on your life. I've had many patients say things like, "I've never thought about it from my dad's point of view. It must have been so hard for him." Such experiences can allow understanding and acceptance to settle in, where that seemed nearly possible before.

5. **Buoyancy.** Sometimes life can make you feel like you're swimming in an ocean. At times, the water is calm and other times you're in the middle of a hurricane. Although ketamine doesn't make the hurricanes go away, it can give you a life jacket. This allows you to start swimming, rather than just feeling like you're drowning all the time. Ketamine can increase your buoyancy so that you can keep your head above water. You still have to swim though. Meaning,

you have to do your part. You have to do the things that you know will improve your mental health and not expect ketamine to do everything for you. It's hard to do that though when the hurricanes are raging and you're just getting swept away.

6. **Life is just better.** Ketamine and psychedelics are not miracle drugs. They don't produce a continuous artificial euphoric state. Some people expect to be on cloud nine all of the time. This is an unrealistic expectation, unfortunately. What I usually see with my patients is that life is similar but just better. It's easier to find the humor in life, to hold down a job, to be there for their family, to feel joy. It doesn't make your problems go away but it can make them easier to navigate and handle.

7. **Letting things go.** My patients frequently report that they are ultra-sensitive to negative situations and have a hard time "letting things go." A negative interaction may cause them to meltdown for hours, days or even weeks at a time. They say that coming in for their ketamine sessions is like putting on a layer of Teflon. It allows negativity to slide off of them in ways that it never could before.

8. **Suicidal thoughts.** Many of my patients struggle with suicidal thoughts on a regular basis. They may not be active, where they have a plan and are determined to implement it. They're usually along the lines of wishing that they could go to sleep and not wake up in the morning. These thoughts can be exhausting to live with. Ketamine can literally make these disappear. This doesn't happen for everyone but most experience a significant reduction in their intensity, frequency, and duration.

Although ketamine helps the majority of my patients, it doesn't help everyone. I really wish that it did. In these cases, patients are almost always grateful that they tried it. When this occurs, I recommend alternative treatment options that would be appropriate for their particular situation.

Finding a ketamine provider

Finding the right ketamine provider for you is paramount. It's one of the key elements of "setting" mentioned above.

Here are a few things that I recommend considering when selecting your ketamine provider:

1. Choose a licensed medical professional.

2. Find a clinic that requires a medical and a psychiatric evaluation. This ensures that ketamine is an appropriate treatment for you from both a medical and psychiatric perspective.

3. Read their reviews online to see what others have to say about them.

4. Ask them if they take your insurance, especially if you're interested in Spravato.

5. See if they offer ketamine-assisted psychotherapy. This is a specialized type of therapy that is done under the influence of ketamine and can increase the efficacy of treatment.[19] You don't have to do it but knowing that it's an option if you do decide you want it is helpful.

6. Trust is everything when it comes to getting ketamine. You'll likely become altered during your sessions and therefore vulnerable. Check out the vibe of the clinic and the staff when you interact with them. If it doesn't feel right, I would look for another place.

Reaching your human potential

There are a number of possible roadblocks that can hinder us from maximizing our human potential. An important one that many overlook is our mental health. I frequently find that my patients have suffered in silence for years before ever seeking help. The reasons for this are varied but many didn't realize that what they were experiencing was actually depression (or another condition). Others were too embarrassed to admit the feelings that they were having to their doctor.

If this is you, addressing these feelings with your medical or mental health provider is the first step. If you suspect that someone you love is struggling, sensitively approaching the topic may be just what they need. I recommend trying traditional treatments first, such as oral antidepressants, to see if they help you. If they fail to provide adequate improvement, looking for a ketamine provider in your area may be the right next step for you or your loved one.

Ketamine and other psychedelics have an incredible ability to reveal what's deep inside of you. What you find is usually a cornucopia of different emotions. As you address the pain and connect to the hope and love that's within you, your path to reaching your human potential will become clearer.

Each ketamine session can reveal new and exciting areas to work on. As you integrate those changes into your life, you'll reap the rewards of your dedicated efforts. It's time to take your future into your capable hands and awaken the glorious person within you. Ketamine may just be the missing tool that you've needed on your journey. Now go and make your beautiful future your new reality.

Notes

[1] Cleveland Clinic. Glutamate. Accessed Jan 12, 2025. https://my.cleve-landclinic.org/health/articles/22839-glutamate

[2] Commissioner, O. of the. (n.d.). *FDA approves new nasal spray medication for treatment-resistant depression; available only at a Certified Doctor's Office or clinic.* U.S. Food and Drug Administration. https://www.fda.gov/news-events/press-announcements/fda-approves-new-nasal-spray-medication-treatment-resistant-depression-available-only-certified

[3] da Costa Gonçalves KT, de Tavares VDO, de Morais Barros ML, de Brito AJC, Cavalcanti-Ribeiro P, Palhano-Fontes F, Falchi-Carvalho M, Arcoverde E, Dos Santos RG, Hallak JEC, de Araujo DB, Galvão-Coelho NL. Ketamine-induced altered states of consciousness: a systematic review of implications for therapeutic outcomes in psychiatric practices. *Eur Arch Psychiatry Clin Neurosci.* 2024 Oct 28. doi: 10.1007/s00406-024-01925-6. Epub ahead of print. PMID: 39467856.

[4] Dai, D., Lacadie, C. M., Holmes, S. E., Cool, R., Anticevic, A., Averill, C., Abdallah, C., & Esterlis, I. (2020). Ketamine normalizes the structural alterations of inferior frontal gyrus in depression. *Chronic Stress, 4.* https://doi.org/10.1177/2470547020980681

[5] Evans, V. D., Arenas, A., Shinozuka, K., Tabaac, B. J., Beutler, B. D., Cherian, K., Fasano, C., & Muir, O. S. (2024). Psychedelic therapy: A Primer for primary care clinicians—ketamine. *American Journal of Therapeutics, 31*(2). https://doi.org/10.1097/mjt.0000000000001721

[6] Ionescu DF, Felicione JM, Gosai A, Cusin C, Shin P, Shapero BG, Deckersbach T. Ketamine-Associated Brain Changes: A Review of the Neuroimaging Literature. *Harv Rev Psychiatry.* 2018 Nov/Dec;26(6):320-339. doi: 10.1097/HRP.0000000000000179. PMID: 29465479; PMCID: PMC6102096.

[7]Kawczak P, Feszak I, Bączek T. Ketamine, Esketamine, and Arketamine: Their Mechanisms of Action and Applications in the Treatment of Depression and Alleviation of Depressive Symptoms. *Biomedicines.* 2024 Oct 9;12(10):2283. doi: 10.3390/biomedicines12102283. PMID: 39457596; PMCID: PMC11505277.

[8] Kohtala S. Ketamine-50 years in use: from anesthesia to rapid antidepressant effects and neurobiological mechanisms. *Pharmacol Rep.* 2021 Apr;73(2):323-345. doi: 10.1007/s43440-021-00232-4. Epub 2021 Feb 20. PMID: 33609274; PMCID: PMC7994242.

[9] Krystal, J. H., Abdallah, C. G., Sanacora, G., Charney, D. S., & Duman, R. S. (2019). Ketamine: A paradigm shift for depression research and treatment. *Neuron, 101*(5), 774—778. https://doi.org/10.1016/j.neuron.2019.02.005

[10] Krystal, J. H., Kavalali, E. T., & Monteggia, L. M. (2023). Ketamine and rapid antidepressant action: New treatments and novel synaptic signaling mechanisms. *Neuropsychopharmacology, 49*(1), 41—50. https://doi.org/10.1038/s41386-023-01629-w

[11] Kumari S, Chaudhry HA, Sagot A, Doumas S, Abdullah H, Alcera E, Solhkhah R, Afzal S. Exploring Esketamine's Therapeutic Outcomes as an FDA-Designated Breakthrough for Treatment-Resistant Depression and Major Depressive Disorder With Suicidal Intent: A Narrative Review. *Cureus.* 2024 Feb 10;16(2):e53987. doi: 10.7759/cureus.53987. PMID: 38476783; PMCID: PMC10928016.

[12] Li, L., & Vlisides, P. E. (2016). Ketamine: 50 years of modulating the mind. *Frontiers in Human Neuroscience, 10.* https://doi.org/10.3389/fnhum.2016.00612

[13] Luscher, B., Feng, M., & Jefferson, S. J. (2020). Antidepressant mechanisms of ketamine: Focus on GABAergic inhibition. *Advances in Pharmacology,* 43—78. https://doi.org/10.1016/bs.apha.2020.03.002

[14] McIntyre, R. S., Alsuwaidan, M., Baune, B. T., Berk, M., Demyttenaere, K., Goldberg, J. F., Gorwood, P., Ho, R., Kasper, S., Kennedy, S. H., Ly-Uson, J., Mansur, R. B., McAllister-Williams, R. H., Murrough, J. W.,

Nemeroff, C. B., Nierenberg, A. A., Rosenblat, J. D., Sanacora, G., Schatzberg, A. F., ... Maj, M. (2023). Treatment-resistant depression: Definition, prevalence, detection, management, and investigational interventions. *World Psychiatry, 22*(3), 394—412. https://doi.org/10.1002/wps.21120

[15] Rădulescu, I., Drăgoi, A., Trifu, S., & Cristea, M. (2021). Neuroplasticity and depression: Rewiring the brain's networks through Pharmacological therapy (review). *Experimental and Therapeutic Medicine, 22*(4). https://doi.org/10.3892/etm.2021.10565

[16] Reed JL, Nugent AC, Furey ML, Szczepanik JE, Evans JW, Zarate CA Jr. Effects of Ketamine on Brain Activity During Emotional Processing: Differential Findings in Depressed Versus Healthy Control Participants. *Biol Psychiatry Cogn Neurosci Neuroimaging.* 2019 Jul;4(7):610-618. doi: 10.1016/j.bpsc.2019.01.005. Epub 2019 Jan 25. PMID: 30826253; PMCID: PMC6612456.

[17] Sahib AK, Loureiro JR, Vasavada M, et al. Modulation of the functional connectome in major depressive disorder by ketamine therapy. *Psychological Medicine.* 2022;52(13):2596-2605. doi:10.1017/S0033291720004560

[18] SPRAVATO® [Prescribing Information]. Titusville, NJ: Janssen Pharmaceuticals, Inc

[19] Yermus, R., Verbora, M., Kennedy, S., McMaster, R., Kratina, S., Wolfson, E., Medrano, B., Bryson, N., Zaer, N., Bottos, J., Setlur, V., & Lo, C. (2023). *Ketamine-Assisted Psychotherapy Provides Lasting and Effective Results in the Treatment of Depression, Anxiety and Post Traumatic Stress Disorder at 3 and 6 Months: Findings from a Large Single-Arm Retrospective Effectiveness Trial.* https://doi.org/10.1101/2023.01.11.23284248

[20] Zanos, P., & Gould, T. D. (2018). Mechanisms of ketamine action as an antidepressant. *Molecular Psychiatry, 23*(4), 801—811. https://doi.org/10.1038/mp.2017.255

[21] Zhang, B., Yang, X., Ye, L., Liu, R., Ye, B., Du, W., Shen, F., Li, Q., Guo, F., Liu, J., Guo, F., Li, Y., Xu, Z., & Liu, Z. (2021). Ketamine activated glutamatergic neurotransmission by GABAergic disinhibition in the medial prefrontal cortex. *Neuropharmacology, 194*, 108382. https://doi.org/10.1016/j.neuropharm.2020.108382

Key takeaways to implement

* Take an honest look at your mental health and if it is hindering you from attaining your human potential, I encourage you to address it.

* If you or someone you love is struggling with mental health challenges and have tried other treatments; consider using the filter above to find an appropriate ketamine provider in your area.

About the author

Growing up in rural Idaho, Greg had dreams of becoming a farmer one day. After getting into college at BYU-Idaho, he decided that he derives more satisfaction from taking care of people, so he became a nurse instead. Upon graduation, he worked in pediatrics, emergency trauma, and directed the Maliheh Free Clinic in Salt Lake City, Utah.

Fluent in Spanish, Greg decided to pursue his graduate degree in nurse anesthesia at the InterAmerican University of Puerto Rico, attracted by both its educational and cultural opportunities. While there, he learned to scuba dive, Latin dance, went skydiving, and fell in love with Puerto Rican food and its people.

His first job as a certified registered nurse anesthetist (CRNA) was just outside of Chicago. He then moved to San Francisco and worked at the University of California, San Francisco. While there, one of his patients told him about the incredible effects that ketamine can have on depression. That pivotal conversation would later inspire him to move to Reno, Nevada, and open Radiance Ketamine Clinic in 2020, followed by Vivid-Life Ketamine Clinic in Concord, California, in 2024.

Greg currently lives in Reno with his fabulous partner, Kiko. When not administering ketamine treatments to his patients, Greg enjoys traveling, gardening, cooking, volunteering, singing in the gay men's chorus, and spending time with those he loves.

www.RadianceKetamineClinic.com   www.VividLifeClinic.com

Part Five

Beyond the Daily Grind

Usha shows us that sexuality is about much more than sex—it's about connecting to the life force energy that makes us feel most alive. Her gentle, practical approach helps us move from disconnection to confidence, from shame to joy. This work transforms not just how we experience pleasure, but how we show up in every area of life.

Usha offers a diverse toolkit for erotic embodiment, much of which transcends conventional notions of sexuality.

— Book momma Chandra

15

Sexually Empowered and Erotically Embodied

Usha Rose

We are sexual beings. Sexual, erotic energy is a potent force that makes the world go round. In truth, it is quite possibly the most powerful energy in the world.

While many might think of eroticism as purely sexual, that is only one expression of it.

To expand beyond that definition, consider all the things that make you feel passionate and alive: dancing your heart out, watching a beautiful sunset, sharing deep emotional experiences or intellectual conversations, making or observing art and music ... the list goes on and on. This is erotic life force energy manifested in your body and your life.

It is the energy that has you dreaming, desiring and creating. It's the energy that has you striving to be a better human, a better partner, parent, boss, or friend.

Having a clear connection, understanding and mastery of your eroticism and sexuality is paramount to living an empowered, full potential life. It will support you to experience greater life satisfaction, freedom and joy.

To gain deeper understanding, mastery and connection to your eroticism and sexuality you need to know how to be present in your body so that you can experience more sensuality, more pleasure and more attunement to the life force energy pulsing through you and all around you.

However, most people are not living this way and therefore cutting themselves short from reaching their human potential.

As busy folks, living life mostly from our heads, with never ending to-do lists, mountains of stress and our faces constantly staring at screens, we rarely slow down enough to be present with sensations in our body, let alone to feel our emotions or listen to the wisdom our bodies have to offer.

It is through our bodies that we can experience tremendous amounts of pleasure, process, heal and move through powerful emotional experiences, and discover some of our most meaningful connections with others.

In recent decades Western science and psychology have started to more fully understand the importance of a mind-body connection, the role of the nervous system and how trauma lives in the body and affects our life.

This has led to a rise in somatic therapy and healing modalities, more interest in Eastern approaches to health and wellness, (like yoga, meditation, Chinese medicine, etc.) and a growing acceptance and field of study in Western cultures on using plant medicines for healing.

As a more holistic approach to health and wellness makes its way to the mainstream, sexuality and eroticism also have a significant place in this conversation, especially if we are interested in discovering our fullest human potential.

Unfortunately, many people live their lives feeling unfulfilled and unsatisfied, cut off from their erotic nature and creative power. They are sexually repressed and shut down, insecure and unhappy.

But it doesn't have to be this way, and I'm honored to offer you five practices to make it super accessible and approachable for you to wake up to your human potential by understanding the value and importance of knowing yourself as a powerfully erotic, sexual being.

Even if you consider yourself a sexually satisfied person, I promise there is more for you to discover here.

To be clear, when I talk about sex, I don't just mean sexual intercourse. I mean sexual energy and eroticism that is available to you regardless of if you are sharing it with another person, multiple people, only yourself, with nature and/or the cosmos.

When you are connected to your own eroticism and come to know yourself as your own best lover, you are already steps ahead of most and on your way to being the most sexually satisfied and alive version of yourself. This will translate into all areas of your life.

Being erotically embodied and sexually empowered extends beyond sensual pleasure, mind-blowing sex and world-shaking orgasms. It affects how you show up in your career and projects, how you show up in relationships with your family, coworkers, community members and partner(s) and how you can choose to move through the world with confidence, generosity and an open heart.

In my career as a Sacred Sexuality Educator and Conscious Relationship Coach I have worked with thousands of clients and students to go from feeling uninspired, sexually disconnected, shutdown and insecure to becoming confident, pleasure-filled, wildly orgasmic, and deeply sexually satisfied.

But this transformation doesn't just improve life in the bedroom, it plays out in all areas of life. You will live more connected to your authentic desires, move from a place of personal power and freedom, attract relationships and opportunities aligned with who you are and create your dream life.

Pleasure and happiness are your birthright. You are capable and worthy of experiencing tremendous sexual satisfaction, pleasure and erotic power. It will support you to live a more fulfilling, inspired, full potential life!

The five practices in this chapter will support you to discover this for yourself.

You may already be on the path of exploring and understanding your sexuality, or this may be new to you. Maybe you've never given it much importance before, or it has been something too taboo to even approach, let alone talk about with someone.

Wherever you are on this path, these practices are going to bring so much more depth, intimacy and inspiration to you, your relationships, your sexuality, and your life.

Practice #1: Develop an intentional self-pleasure practice

An intentional self-pleasure practice is essential to deepening intimacy with yourself and becoming more aware of the wisdom of your body. It supports your ability to stay present and enhances your sensitivity to the pleasurable sensations of your body.

Through this practice you are cultivating and nourishing the most important relationship you have: your relationship with yourself.

It is a simple practice of setting aside intentional time to be lovingly present with yourself and aware of your physical sensations using the three Tantric keys for moving energy: breath, sound, and movement.

In case you are wondering if I am talking about masturbation, let me explain.

The reason I use the term self-pleasuring instead of masturbation is because most people think of masturbation as genital stimulation with an intended goal of orgasm. While that is also a lovely practice, I'm talking about something beyond that.

A self-pleasure practice can be sexual and include the genitals and orgasms, but that is not the focus. The focus is on cultivating the ability to stay present in your body, enhance sensitivity, and infuse your body, mind, and nervous system with positive, healing intentions.

For example, you might set the intention to feel more loving and accepting of your body or experience a greater sense of safety in your body.

Honor your self-pleasuring practice as a sacred and special time by mindfully setting the space. Find a private space to be with yourself, clear all distractions, light candles, put on music, and set an intention for your practice.

This is your time to be present with yourself and to enjoy your own company. Here is one idea of how you might do this, but feel free to improvise and be creative.

While lying down or standing up, take a few deep breaths, relaxing and feeling your body, your breath, and any physical sensations. Move, stretch, and shake your body, allowing it to move any way that feels good. Take some deep breaths with attention on your pelvis and genitals and let out some sound. Touch your entire body in whatever way feels good to you. Caress your face, stroke your arms and legs, massage your breasts. If you include genital touch, explore new ways of touching and notice if you fall into old patterns. Stay present with all sensations. Let out sounds, moans, and sighs. Allow yourself to be uninhibited, curious, playful, sensual, sexual.

If your mind begins to wander, bring it back gently, without shame or judgment, to the present moment, to the body, to sensations. Cultivate feelings of self-appreciation, self-love, and gratitude.

The goal is not to reach any specific state of arousal or orgasm, but to stay present.

As you do this practice you might find that memories, heavy thoughts or emotions arise, like grief, anger, resistance, or self-doubt. Try not to judge or push them away. Instead invite them to move, be expressed and released using breath, sound and movement. Cultivate the qualities of acceptance, self-love, compassion and patience with yourself.

This practice is tremendously healing and will positively shift your relationship to your body, emotions, and sexuality so that you feel more whole and empowered.

Other ideas for a sensual self-pleasure practice include giving yourself a full body oil massage, taking a hot bubble bath with presence on sensuality, put on sexy lingerie and dance for yourself erotically, spend intentional time in nature activating *all* your senses: sight, sound, smell, touch and taste!

Action Steps:

- Self-Pleasure for at least five minutes every morning before you get out of bed. Use the ideas listed above for inspiration.

- Place your hands somewhere comforting on your body and say out loud at least five things you love and appreciate about yourself, your body, and your sexuality. Do this every day. Bonus points for doing it while looking in a mirror.

- Use my free video for a guided, sensual, self-breast massage practice here: www.usharose.com/selfbreastmassage

Practice #2: Dance, play and move your body freely

Dancing, playing and moving your body freely supports you in reducing inhibitions and insecurities so that you become more comfortable and confident in your body. This will serve you to become more sexually confident and discover more freedom to sexually express yourself.

Physically moving your body helps move all sorts of energy (mental, emotional, physical, sexual). It gets you out of your head, present in your body and connected to the erotic life force always present within you. This is key for being able to expand your sensuality and pleasure potential.

While exercise is important for confidence, health and feeling good, it is also important to play and move your body authentically to develop your ability and comfort with expressing yourself.

Many people struggle to embody their erotic nature because they feel self-conscious, insecure or shy. To shift that I urge you to tip-toe out of your comfort zone and lean into those uncomfortable edges.

Practice moving your body with curiosity, playfulness, creativity, spontaneity, and authentic expression. Let yourself be silly, awkward, and weird. The less you take yourself so seriously, the more ease, comfort and confidence you will have to express yourself sexually.

Forgot how to play?

Unfortunately, most adults don't play enough. Some ways of playing include, most obviously, spending time with children and really diving into their world. Go along with their make-believe stories and adventures, adding your own imagination and creativity.

Another way is to get out in nature and become a curious explorer of your environment as if you're an alien from another planet discovering earth for the first time. Interact with your surroundings with childlike curiosity and wonder. Touch and smell the flowers, crawl around on rocks, hug and talk with the trees, splash around in the waves and roll in the sand.

Another great playful exercise to release inhibitions and become less self-conscious is to get together with some friends (of all ages) and interact with each other while embodying different animals. Flap your arms like wings and screech like a bird, leap around like slimy frogs, wrestle and tumble over each other like puppies and scratch and sniff each other like wild monkeys. The more ridiculous you feel the better you know it is working to release your inhibitions and lighten up your ideas of yourself.

Think you don't know how to dance?

If you are completely new to dancing, there are a few different ways to get started. The first and most obvious of course, is to just dance! Put on some music at home that inspires and arouses your erotic energy and get moving!

If dancing is really an edge for you, try a structured dance class that inspires you, like partner dance, belly dance, modern, or African. Having guidance and learning something new will stretch your comfort zone and give you encouragement, resilience and confidence in your body's ability to move in new ways. If you feel intimidated in groups, start with a private lesson!

The third way, which is my favorite, is to find a free-form conscious dance practice like Ecstatic Dance, 5Rhythms, Contact Improv, or Soul-Motion where you will be invited and welcomed to dance unstructured. Here you are encouraged to move your body anyway you want with total freedom to creatively express yourself. This will definitely help reduce your inhibitions.

Action steps:

- Create a playlist that inspires and arouses your erotic energy, then dance to it!

- Find a dance class or conscious dance event and go to it!

- Dance at least once a week with the intention of being in touch with your sensuality and erotic nature. Focus on movements that feel erotic, touch yourself sensually and even dress in a way that makes you feel sexy. Try stripping!

- Get some friends together to explore nature and play the animal embodiment game described above.

Practice #3: Educate yourself about your erotic nature

Your brain is the most important sexual organ! Therefore, knowing and understanding your sexuality is foundational to being in your power.

To discover who you are as a sexual being helps to educate yourself about eroticism. Learn how your body and mind work erotically so you understand what turns you on and turns you off.

There are many resources for educating yourself about sexual anatomy, arousal, and eroticism — from books, to podcasts, to workshops, to working with a wide range of professionals who specialize in the field of sexuality. Additionally, research indicates that talking about our sexuality with others greatly improves our sexual health and makes us feel more empowered.

Connect with close friends or lovers and talk about sex! This is a great way to gather and share information, experiences, support, and resources. It also helps you to normalize and accept your sexuality. No matter how you are feeling in your sexual exploration: frustrated, confused, inspired, hopeful, lost ... you are not alone. Other people are going through similar experiences. If you don't have trusted friends to discuss this, seek out a professional who can support you in your sexual exploration.

Knowing and understanding yourself and your lovers sexually gives you power. Living in your sexual power gives you confidence and freedom to express yourself, to move towards what you want, to experience greater satisfaction, and to live a life you love.

Action steps:

- Read books, listen to podcasts, and seek out educational content about sexuality.

- Take a workshop, retreat, or training program that specifically relates to sexuality.

- Start talking about sexuality with trusted friends. Get a group going where you can discuss and share experiences, resources, and information.

- Book a session with a professional who will support you in exploring your erotic nature.

Practice #4: Get in touch with your desires!

If you want to live a full potential life you love, a life you are powerfully creating for yourself, it's necessary to get in touch with your desires!

Desire is creative fuel. It guides and inspires us towards what we want.

When we know what we want we can make clear, aligned decisions that lead us towards our desires. This is a very powerful way to create the life you dream of and live from a place of happiness, gratitude, and joy.

When we don't know what we want, we can be like a leaf blowing in the wind, allowing resentment and dissatisfaction to brew.

Erotic energy is the creative life force within us. The more we connect with our desires, the more energy we bring to our sexuality and the greater our ability to create what we want in life. Desire and erotic energy work together as powerful creative resources, fueling passion and vitality.

So how do you know what you want?

Oftentimes I find in my coaching practice that many clients don't know what they want.

If this is true for you, it can be helpful to start by asking yourself "What DON'T I want?" Or "What am I afraid of?" From there you can start to explore what you DO want, based on knowing what you don't want!

Ultimately what everyone wants is to feel good, be happy, and live a satisfying life. Notice the key thing in this statement of what we all want is a FEELING! Not a thing.

Many people can get caught up thinking about the things we want, like a nicer house, more money, an amazing partner, a vacation, or a better body ... but why do we want those things? We want those things because we think those things will make us feel good.

What we really want is the *feeling* we hope those things will create.

We want a nicer house because we think it will make us feel more peaceful and happy.

We want more money because we believe it will provide feelings of freedom and security.

We want an amazing partner to feel more love and happiness.

We want a vacation because we think it will bring us feelings of relaxation and enjoyment.

We want a better body to feel more confident and healthy.

But the truth is, no THING can reliably make us happy.

We might have all the things we want, but none of the good feelings that go with them. So, what to do?

Focus on how you want to feel! Go after the feelings, not the things. This is where our desire guides us! When we stay focused on the feeling we desire as our internal compass, we choose the things based on, "How does this make me feel? Does this thing, this decision, this action bring me joy?" If yes, then go for it! If not, then choose something else.

Easier said than done, I know. That's because we have not been taught to live this way, especially those who grew up as girls and were conditioned to become people-pleasing women, putting others' needs before our own. This can be a hard pattern to break and requires the ability to say no.

This is something I work with *a lot* with my clients. Claiming our desires, feeling worthy of them and developing strong boundaries are essential to be able to powerfully choose what is aligned with our truth.

Along those same lines, we need to have courage and be able to trust our internal compass, even if it doesn't make logical sense.

This can be challenging at first, but when we start choosing and living in this way, magic starts to happen. New opportunities start to emerge, and life unfolds in unexpected ways.

Knowing what we want in life, also applies to knowing what we want sexually. As discussed in the previous chapter, educating yourself about your eroticism is one part of discovering that, and the other part is experimentation.

The key qualities to bring to experimentation are curiosity and playfulness, which is why learning how to play and getting comfortable and confident in your body is so important.

It's important to explore with an open mind but make sure you are staying in your power and in your choice. Go slow with new explorations. The more present you are, the more connected you can be to your sensations, and the more aware, clear, and sensitive you can be with your boundaries!

Action steps:

- Get out a journal and ask yourself these questions: "What don't I want?" Or "What am I afraid of?" This can help you identify obstacles and limiting beliefs that may be holding you back. Next ask yourself: "What do I want?" Write down anything and everything that comes to you. Dream big. Anything is possible. Don't limit yourself based on what you think is possible. Let your imagination have free reign for this exercise, even if you discover contradictory desires. This supports new insights, positive emotions and aspirations.

- Every morning ask yourself, "How do I want to feel today?" Take some time to embody your desired feeling. Allow this desired feeling to be your compass for the rest of the day, moving you toward that which makes you feel good.

- Practice asking for what you want and saying no. Get courageous voicing your desires and boundaries with confidence and certainty. Take any opportunity to claim your desire, from simply stating your order at a restaurant, picking what movie you want to watch, to boldly telling your lover what you want in the bedroom. Like a muscle, this skill can take some practice to strengthen, but it is essential for living a full potential life of happiness and fulfillment.

Practice #5: Use your erotic energy for transformation and manifestation, i.e. Sex Magic!

As previously discussed, erotic energy is the energy of creation. When we channel that energy with positive intention towards what we want, we give that desire more creative life force and power. As many believe in prayer or intention setting, our thoughts and words have power, and when we combine those words, prayers or intentions with erotic energy we can make magic!

Let me explain.

As mentioned earlier, our nervous system is an important piece of the puzzle when it comes to healing. It is also a vital component in our ability to experience sexual satisfaction. That's because it needs to be relaxed, trusting that you are safe, in order to experience pleasure.

Your brain, the most important sexual organ, is wired to keep you safe and is constantly scanning for danger. Unconsciously, anything unknown or unfamiliar often registers as a potential threat.

Therefore, we need to teach our brains and rewire our nervous system to believe and trust that our desires are not only safe to have and experience, but also pleasurable. We do this by entering into altered states of consciousness so that all parts of the brain and nervous system are activated, and then imagining or envisioning the experience that we desire. The mind does not know the difference between imagination and reality; thus, we are creating new neural pathways and embodied beliefs that the desired experience we are imagining is pleasurable and safe.

One of the ways we can get into an altered state of consciousness is through heightened states of pleasure, arousal, or orgasm. Other ways, such as dance, music, breathwork, prayer, and medicine work have been used since ancient times for the purpose of healing, connecting to Spirit, and channeling intuitive wisdom.

Affirmations related to claiming your desires only access the prefrontal cortex. Combining affirmations, a clear vision, and congruent emotions while in an altered state amplifies your effectiveness in shifting beliefs, clearing unconscious blocks, and aligning your actions with your desires.

In order for the practice of using your erotic energy for transformation and manifestation to be effective you need to know what you want, so make sure you've spent some time with practice #4 first! Then follow the steps for creating a powerful sex magic ritual for yourself.

You might use this practice for manifesting your dream job, more money, next home or ideal partner, but remember it is not so much about the specific *thing* of your desire, but about the experience. So, imagine how it will *feel* having this desire manifested, and then trust in the universe to deliver whatever is in highest alignment for you and all beings. It might not be that specific car or job, but you will manifest the security and satisfaction that you imagine having because of that thing.

To say it a different way, use this practice for transforming your identity, meaning to become the best version of yourself that you can imagine.

What does your life look like when you are living as your fullest potential self? What are the embodied feelings you want to move through life with?

Is it confidence, power, joy, freedom, security?

Imagine yourself as the most radiant, sexy, outgoing, creative, successful version of yourself while in intentional, prayerful states of altered consciousness and you will start living, moving and experiencing yourself as exactly that. So, get clear on *who* and *how* you want to *be* in the world and use this practice as often as you like in order to live your fullest potential version of yourself.

7 Steps to a Sex Magic ritual

1. Get crystal clear on your desire. What are you wanting to manifest, heal or transform? Write it down and speak it out loud.

2. Spend time imagining having this desire. Visualize it with ALL of your senses. What do you see, smell, feel, taste and hear that lets you know you have achieved this desire?

3. How do you FEEL having this desire? Begin to embody those high vibe feeling states right now. (Example, feeling relaxed, happy, confident, secure, free, safe, joyful, etc.)

4. Bring yourself into a heightened state of pleasure and arousal. Touch and pleasure yourself, move your body, make sound, and turn yourself on.

5. Send that pleasurable energy all over your body, charging your chakras and visualizing the manifestation of your desire.

6. While orgasming, or at the peak of your arousal and pleasure, visualize your desire and embody the feeling state of having that desire.

7. Send your orgasmic energy coupled with your vision and/or prayer off into the universe trusting it will become manifested/transformed as it is in alignment with your highest good and the highest good of all beings.

Complete this practice by resting in trust and surrender, continuing to visualize and embody the feelings of having your desires. Let your body, mind, and heart be nourished by your presence and pleasure.

Note: This practice can be done solo or with a lover. You can share your intention with your lover, collaborate on a shared desire and practice sex magic together, or keep it all to yourself: it's totally up to you.

Remember that whenever you are practicing magic to add the addendum after your intention: "As it is in alignment with the highest good of all beings!" And as one of my favorite teachers likes to say, "This or something even better!"

If you're ready to live a more erotically embodied, sexually empowered life so that you can reach your greatest human potential, I hope you'll experiment with these practices and see your life transform.

Your erotic life force is already within you, waiting to be awakened. Each small step you take toward presence and authenticity is an act of reclaiming your power. Trust your body's wisdom, honor your desires, and watch as this energy transforms every area of your life.

Key takeaways to implement

Ready to begin your journey toward sexual empowerment and erotic embodiment? Here are simple, powerful actions you can take right now to start connecting with your fullest potential:

* Start Your Morning with Presence:

    Before getting out of bed tomorrow, spend 5 minutes with your hands on your body (heart, belly, or anywhere that feels comforting). Take deep breaths and simply notice physical sensations. This begins building your body awareness and presence — the foundation of all erotic embodiment.

* Dance to One Song:

    Put on a song that makes you feel alive and move your body freely for 3-4 minutes. Don't worry about looking good — focus on how it feels to move authentically. This immediately gets you out of your head and into your body's wisdom.

* Ask Yourself: "How Do I Want to Feel Today?":

    Right now, pause and ask this question. Choose one feeling state (confident, joyful, free, sensual) and take three actions throughout your day that align with that desired feeling. This is to practice using *desire* as your internal compass.

* Set One Clear Boundary:

    Practice saying "no" to something today that doesn't align with how you want to feel, or say "yes" to something you truly desire. This could be as simple as choosing what to eat for dinner or declining an invitation that drains you. Every small choice builds your sovereignty.

＊ End Your Day with a Celebration:

Before sleep, place your hands somewhere comforting on your body and acknowledge yourself for taking steps toward living more fully. Appreciation for your courage creates positive momentum for continued growth.

About the author

Usha Rose is the founder of the Erotic Embodiment Institute and a Facilitator for the International School of Temple Arts. As a VITA certified Sexual Empowerment & Conscious Relationship Coach, she is passionate about supporting her clients and students to live more sexually confident, sensually embodied, pleasure-based lives so that they can powerfully create the most nourishing and satisfying relationships, career, and life possible.

You can access her free resources, learn more about her online coaching and courses, and check out her in-person trainings by visiting her website:

www.usharose.com

Maria challenges aging norms by building muscle and increasing stability. She exemplifies the possibility of questioning conventional wisdom about physical decline with age, showing us that vitality can continue and even increase throughout our later years.

When I encounter someone with exceptional vitality, I ask for their top health hack. She looks much younger than she actually is.

— *Book momma Chandra*

16

Gaining Vitality while Reimagining Aging

Dr. Maria Cristina Sheehan

Aging is a journey we all share, an experience that ties us together across different walks of life. Yet, too often, aging is viewed through a negative lens, full of fear and loss. In this chapter, I aim to shift that perspective and shine a light on your potential at every age, challenging the stereotypes that often obscure the aging process.

Aging is an opportunity for growth and self-discovery, not a decline. I want you to question the societal narrative that aging equals inevitable deterioration and present a more empowering view of aging as a time for continued growth, achievement, and vitality.

I'll explore the science of aging and debunk common myths — by sharing stories of inspiring individuals who have defied age-related stereotypes. I'll show you the power of mindset in shaping how aging is experienced, as well as touch on the importance of physical and mental fitness in promoting healthy aging.

By challenging these stereotypes, you can unlock a new understanding of human potential that doesn't diminish with age but continues to evolve. Your potential is more than understanding aging — it's about changing how you see it.

Myths of aging

I find myself in a society that often whispers, and sometimes shouts, that aging means inevitable physical decline. And people around me seem to accept it without reason. They expect their futures to be graced by frailty and a steady withdrawal from the healthy and fun activities that once brought joy and vitality. However, I stand, or instead jog, in firm opposition to this notion. Physical deterioration is not a foregone conclusion of aging; it is a challenge that can be met with determination, knowledge, and a proactive lifestyle.

Many people view physical deterioration as an expected aspect of aging. What if you challenge this assumption? According to the writers, Crowley and Lodge, of *Younger Next Year,* around 70 percent of the average aging process after 50 is not biologically essential but is influenced by lifestyle choices. The belief is that with the correct lifestyle changes, half of the illnesses and serious accidents that older individuals are likely to experience can be eliminated. This concept was transformative for me since it suggested that my older years could be a time of rejuvenation rather than a steady decline.

Recent advances in the science of aging tell us that the human body is much more adaptable. Science now understands that, on a cellular level, one can greatly influence the biological processes. Regular physical activity, emotional well-being, and a balanced diet sends signals to the body that can actually reverse signs of decline. This isn't just wishful thinking — it's backed by science.

One of the most critical aspects in fighting physical decline is exercise, not simply strolling but engaging in activities that challenge our perceptions of what we are capable of as we age. Resistance exercise and strength sports such as cycling, tennis, and skiing are not limited to the young. They are necessary for preserving muscle mass, boosting metabolism, and improving cognitive function. I started strength training at age 69, and I can attest to this fact that strength and muscle mass can be built beautifully with consistent effort.

Personal experiences often speak louder than theoretical knowledge. I often feel astonished and re-energized by the physical capabilities I've developed. My trainer often reminds me of where we started eight years ago. To build muscle mass you have to increase the load or amount of weight lifted or pulled over time. That's exactly what I did. Starting slowly and ending strong is the way to go, demonstrating the strength that can be developed and maintained even as we age. Recently, he introduced me to a modified stiff-leg deadlift. Initially daunting, this exercise quickly became feasible as my body adapted to the new challenge. Pulling 95 pounds when I weigh only 120 pounds was not something I would have imagined doing a decade ago.

Tao Porchon-Lynch, who taught yoga until her passing at 101, embodies the vitality that can be sustained through a lifelong dedication to physical and mental wellness. She was recognized as the world's oldest yoga teacher, a title that speaks volumes about her health and agility. Tao's life was a vibrant tapestry of dance, yoga, and activism, which kept her mind sharp and her spirit youthful. Her practice and yoga teaching, which she continued diligently throughout her life, contributed significantly to her cognitive and physical stamina. Her ability to perform complex yoga poses and teach with such enthusiasm at her age powerfully counters the myth of inevitable physical and cognitive decline.

Similarly, Eileen Kramer is an extraordinary example of enduring creativity and intellect. At 105, she wrote a book and, as of her last interview at 108, was still engaged in the creative arts; she is living proof of the cognitive capacities that can be maintained through creative engagement. Eileen danced and continued to choreograph and perform, illustrating that cognitive engagement through the arts can profoundly impact maintaining mental acuity. Her creative work showcased her cognitive abilities and highlighted her physical strength and balance, challenging the misconceptions about aging and physical activity.

Aging with vigor

These examples of Tao Porchon-Lynch and Eileen Kramer offer more than inspiration —   they provide a blueprint for aging gracefully with vigor. They show that engaging in physical activities like yoga and dance maintains and can enhance our physical capabilities. Moreover, their stories emphasize the importance of pursuing passions and continuing to learn, grow, and contribute, which are vital for cognitive health.

Dr. Gabrielle Lyon, the author of *Forever Strong,* argues compellingly that every individual over 40 needs to engage in strength training to age energetically. This resonates deeply with my practices and the visible benefits I've reaped from prioritizing physical strength. Dr. Lyon emphasizes that skeletal muscle acts as a locomotor organ and a metabolic regulator, crucial for managing blood sugars, fats, and overall physical resilience. The development and maintenance of muscle mass through strength training are pivotal for mobility and stability and as a preventative measure against numerous age-related health issues.

Engaging in regular strength training has been transformative for me. It has enhanced my physical capabilities and boosted my confidence in my ability to adapt and embrace new challenges. Dr. Lyon also highlights the necessity of maximizing protein intake, advocating for a diet that supports muscle repair and growth. This approach ensures that our bodies are better equipped to handle the stresses of aging, with robust musculature supporting a more active and engaged lifestyle.

The idea that we are too old to change dismisses the remarkable adaptability of the human body and spirit. Throughout my 70s, I have adopted new routines, learned new skills, and made significant lifestyle changes that have profoundly affected my quality of life. Whether adjusting dietary habits to include more protein or adopting a new exercise regimen, these changes are feasible and beneficial at any age.

We often hear that our muscles dictate the chemistry of growth throughout our bodies, and it is through exercise that these positive changes are set in motion. Improved sleep, weight management, and resistance to diseases like arthritis and even Alzheimer's can all stem from maintaining an active lifestyle. The journey into older age can be one of growth rather than decay if we choose to live actively.

Questioning inevitable cognitive decline

Leading neuroscientist Dr. Daniel Amen strongly opposes the idea that cognitive decline must accompany aging. His research has been instrumental in illustrating how various interventions can not only prevent but also reverse signs of brain aging. This has profound implications for us as we age, suggesting that our mental faculties can be preserved and even enhanced.

What stands out in Dr. Amen's findings is the impact of daily choices on brain health. It's not just about doing crossword puzzles or reading books; it's about holistic health management, including diet, physical exercise, stress reduction, and maintaining a healthy sleep schedule. For example, maintaining a healthy weight, engaging in regular physical activities, and ensuring adequate sleep are fundamental to keeping cognitive functions sharp.

On a personal note, I have incorporated several of Dr. Amen's recommendations into my daily routine. I ensure that I engage in strength training and cardiovascular exercises, which are good for my body and essential for my brain health. Limiting alcohol consumption, focusing on a diet rich in omega-3 fatty acids and antioxidants, as well as a diet low in processed foods—all support my brain's needs to function optimally.

Another aspect of maintaining cognitive function is social engagement. Positive relationships stimulate one's brain through emotional and intellectual exchanges. I make it a point to engage with my community, participate in group activities, and maintain close connections with family and friends. These social interactions provide emotional support and contribute to a positive mental state, which is crucial for mental agility.

Dr. Sara Gottfried's work on genetic predispositions to diseases underscores the importance of proactive health management. Her recommendations for taking supplements like CoQ10 and engaging in new learning endeavors are particularly resonant. I am working on improving my foreign language skills and relearning how to play the piano — which I haven't touched since childhood. I have been studying yoga and mastering complex poses and just started taking gymnastics classes. This keeps my mind engaged and ensures that my brain remains in a state of growth and adaptability.

Positive stress

Dr. David Sinclair promotes the idea of maintaining a slight caloric restriction. Staying a little hungry is not about deprivation; rather, it's about avoiding the overconsumption that often leads to metabolic and cellular stress. This approach is rooted in the principle that minor stress on the body, like that from lower calorie intake, can enhance resilience and vitality.

He also advocates for the benefits of hot and cold therapies. Regular use of saunas and cold showers can stimulate the body's stress response, improving circulation, reducing inflammation, and activating longevity genes. Once integrated into daily routines, these practices can enhance overall cellular function and longevity.

Another key aspect of Dr. Sinclair's approach includes using supplements like Nicotinamide Mononucleotide (NMN) and resveratrol. NMN is a precursor to NAD+ (nicotinamide adenine dinucleotide), a critical coenzyme in the body that declines with age. Resveratrol, found naturally in the skins of grapes and berries, has been noted for its anti-aging properties, particularly in activating sirtuins, a group of proteins involved in cellular health and longevity.

Echoing these sentiments, Dr. Michael Merzenich, a pioneer in neuroplasticity, discusses how our life choices can actively degrade or improve our brain functioning. His concept of "brain plasticity rules" emphasizes the need for various brain-engaging activities that challenge the mind and body. This aligns with my own experiences, as I find that varying my exercises and introducing new challenges has kept my body healthy and sharpened my cognitive abilities.

New habits

Adopting new habits in one's 70s can be challenging but far from impossible. The key lies in making a committed decision, seeking the right information, and getting support where needed. Health coaches, trainers specialized in senior fitness, and community groups can provide encouragement and guidance essential for sustaining these changes.

Contrary to the myth, aging can be a time of reinvention and renewal. I've witnessed peers taking up new hobbies like painting, starting yoga, or even entering athletic competitions well into their later years. These stories are not just inspiring; they are clear evidence that change is possible and enriching at any age.

How to maximize fitness regardless of age: Brain and body

There is no ceiling on your ability to maintain fitness and enhance your human potential, but embracing a simple protocol is essential to do so. Your brain requires everything your body requires to launch yourself into healthy final decades of life. What you do for your body you do for your brain and vice versa.

Your mindset is powerfully navigating how you age. The first step is to increase your belief in what is possible in regard to cognitive acuity and physical ability. Lack of this belief will inevitably produce decline. Eliminating stress and negative thoughts by meditation and listening to motivational videos is a place to start. Just a few minutes a day sitting in silence calming the mind and viewing life through a positive lens is what I do every day. It takes practice but well worth the effort.

Taking the first step to building muscle mass regardless of age is the second step. The benefits have already been discussed but cannot be stressed enough. It is not true that at any point in life it's too late to begin. There even have been studies on centenarians noting that they could build back a bit of muscle mass using light weights.

Finally eliminating as much sugar as possible and as quickly as possible is a protocol to embrace. I've become a label reading detective only because sugar and all of its sneaky aliases reside in nearly every packaged food that we consume. If you want to age faster, then do not heed this advice. We live in a world with overly processed artificial ingredients in our foods. If you don't recognize an ingredient don't purchase that food. Flour in the US is ultra processed causing inflammation, gut issues, and early aging. Sadly, we cannot trust most of the bread on our grocery shelves to be beneficial to your health.

I also recognize alcohol as a toxin injurious to my body and aging me more quickly. So my final tip is: drink occasionally, seldom, or never if you can.

Your vibrant potential is designed to be within you until your last breath. Adopt a protocol to ensure that every day is one of great health leading to lifelong potential.

Key takeaways to implement

* Believe that elevating your health is possible as you age.

* Start lifting weights and engage in a variety of exercises. I have videos for age related strength training on my website: drmariacristina.com

* Limit your sugar, highly processed foods, and alcohol.

About the author

Dr. Maria Cristina, Sheehan Health and Wellness, is a health and wellness educator and expert in transforming aging as we know it.

Her academic degrees include two master's degrees and a doctorate, and she holds certifications as a personal trainer and health coach. She served 20 years as a college president prior to her wellness journey.

She has been featured on the Aging and Awesome TV series and is a requested speaker for audiences wishing to improve their health and turn back time. She is a natural body fitness competitor winning multiple gold and silver medals in international competitions since 2017.

As a speaker she enjoys motivating college and university faculty and staff by providing keynotes for wellness weeks and providing customized wellness workshops for administrators and their teams.

drmariacristina.com

Britta radiates magical dynamism in both her life and coaching practice. Her electrifying energy and dedication to personal growth are inspirational. Her coaching creates a rare balance of vulnerability and empowerment that catalyzes authentic transformation.

From soul-led living to navigating life's most challenging marriage decisions, Britta is an invaluable ally on the journey to authenticity.

— Book momma Chandra

17

Create a Soul-Led Life

Britta Jo

This is a new age — a time ripe with possibilities to expand human potential both individually and collectively, and we see the awakening happening all around us. Those who just one or two generations ago would have lived lives of standard growth are experiencing shifts of multiple lifetimes condensed into one. It is an exciting and overwhelming time.

Our nervous systems, built for the old ways of limited growth over one lifetime, are being stretched and at times overwhelmed by so much change in such a short time. This amount of growth is a lot for one human psyche to handle.

Where in the past, we have pushed and pressured or strived and achieved as a society, these very actions now burn us out. We see more and more disillusionment with the status quo. More people are asking, "Why am I here? Does any of this matter?" and less are accepting old truths or blindly getting back in line. More are longing for lives that are deeply meaningful both individually and collectively, and less are willing to live lives spent only in service of the greater good.

No longer can we be content with the either/or of old. We are ready to live lives filled with *both*, both individual fulfillment AND collective ascendance. Lives that I call *Soul-Led*.

To make this leap is no small task. It requires transmutation; the act of individuals alchemizing their personal suffering and trauma into love and consciousness instead. These individuals help usher us as a species across this next threshold of expanded human potential.

Five beliefs to support your journey

In my work with women considering divorce, I see repeatedly how those who are chosen for these transmutational lives are often called by deep, unrelenting, and powerful *soul calls*. Over the years I have been fascinated by what beliefs allow them to make these shifts. Shifts into lives that perhaps look nothing like what people had predicted for themselves, but feel undeniably more aligned with their inner knowing.

In this chapter, I will share five beliefs I have identified that facilitate living a truly soul-led life. Each of these beliefs can help you release judgment and control and surrender with love to the potential your life has in store for you if you embrace your soul-led journey.

As you read each belief, I recommend you metaphorically hold and examine it while noticing where it lands in your body and heart. If it doesn't resonate, let it go. For the ones that do resonate, take care, plant them deeply in your garden of beliefs and they will sustain you in ways you cannot imagine for your epic soul journey ahead.

Belief #1: Your current life is only one part of your soul journey

As I've searched for answers concerning what we're doing here, I've come across a theme that resonates with me around the concept that "this life is a dream," meaning that each person's current human life is only a part of their soul's journey. If you allow your mind to entertain that it is only one part, then your mind can zoom out and wonder: what if we are here to learn and grow; what if we choose our challenges and sign up for our experiences? Then we can let go of the urge to control and dictate everything with such fear of the future. Rather, just like in a dream, we are here for the experience; when it is all over, no one is truly hurt, destroyed, or damaged because it all unfolds and is part of our soul's journey.

If you have read the book "Journey of Souls," you will have a general idea of this concept. If you haven't read the book you can imagine each soul choosing their body, their life, and the general challenges; meaning each soul signs up for going to school on Earth. A stretch? For sure, just like all ideas about why we are truly here, including the ones accepted by millions in the major religions.

Thus, I invite you to suspend your disbelief during this chapter and open instead to curiosity about what else could be. The more we learn about quantum theory and how time and space do not follow our previously conceived rules, the more I find peace in admitting how much none of us truly knows. Even extending to the idea that perhaps we all are experiencing some form of soul amnesia when we are born.

With that said, I want to share a personal experience I had that took these concepts I was learning mentally and showed me how they could be verified through the body's "inner knowings" as well.

In 2021, my mother passed away from pancreatic cancer. The years leading up to her death were rocky for us. I started therapy in 2017, learned about and identified narcissistic personality disorder behaviors in her, and dramatically limited my contact with her. When she passed away, I felt relief rather than grief. A person with whom I had so much pain and ongoing uneasiness around was now gone and I was free.

With this as my main sentiment around her death, I was deeply surprised when on a beautiful summer evening two months after her funeral she visited me in spirit. This was not something I had ever experienced before nor sought out or hoped for.

To set the scene, I was alone out in my barn that evening with my favorite classical composer playing on a speaker as I danced in the dark and processed waves of joy and love for my life that were coming in at that moment when I suddenly felt a presence enter the barn behind me. I knew instantaneously that it was she as she came up behind me and wrapped her arms around me in a hug.

At that moment, 33 years of pain and hurt were wiped away in an instant as I felt the impact of the clarity and purity of her love. It felt like seeing her, truly seeing HER, without all of her pain and trauma and internal demons, for the very first time. In addition, the love I felt from her in that moment was indescribable.

It is hard for words to convey what it is like to feel disconnected and energetically confused by your mother your entire life and then to in one moment have this flash of clarity where you finally realize, "Oh she did love me. She loved me so deeply; I just could not feel it because her unprocessed trauma and pain blocked her from me. It was never about me not being lovable; it was about her not being able to convey love due to her pain."

It was one of the biggest healing moments of my life and with all the reading I had been doing around the idea that your current life is just one part of your soul's journey, this piece of the puzzle clicked into place for me.

If this life is just one part, then of course there could be moments like this after death where, just like when you wake up from a dream, you realize, "What I thought was going on and seemed so important actually wasn't the whole story, there was more here than what I could realize while in the dream." That was what I felt with my mother that night. I wouldn't believe it if I hadn't experienced it myself; that so much acquired pain, disconnection, confusion, and trauma could be wiped out from the past in an instant.

This is the clearest way I know of making sense of the amount of suffering that happens in the world and the apparent injustices of it all. The Mormon theology I was raised with suggests this life is your one shot at reaching heaven. It never sat well with me that if a God that supposedly loves us created us, he would let so many hurt and suffer in this life and that be it, their one shot. Could there instead be something far greater than we can imagine going on here? Opening to that possibility is one of the quickest ways to embark on a more expansive soul-led trajectory for your life.

Belief #2: You cannot mess this up; your path is already planned and unfolding perfectly

About midway through my journey uncovering these beliefs, I had gotten into the idea of manifestation, i.e., intentionally picking and visualizing what you want and then calling it in. I invested a lot of time and energy in this approach only to learn repeatedly that the reality (was) ... I am not in control.

What I was trying to manifest (especially if I was super specific about what it should look like) would *not* show up and instead, my life would often have unexpected left turns. These could be intensely disorienting and painful when I was caught up in the illusion that what I had wanted to happen was what was supposed to and thus something was now going wrong.

Eventually, I learned that the answer was not to keep fighting for what *I* wanted, but to surrender to life and in the words of Matt Kahn, "Love what is." The more I learned how to surrender into these twists and turns and believe I was safe regardless, the more I began tapping into this "peace that surpasses all understanding."

To help wrap your mind around this belief, I want to provide the framework that I pieced together from various concepts I had learned.

To start, in the belief of this being "one part of your soul's journey," I mentioned how time and space are relative. The best example I have seen of this would be in the movies *Interstellar* and *Everything, Everywhere, All At Once*. This coupled with various references through my many readings to a *higher-self* led me to resonate most with an idea found in "The Definitive Book of Human Design" which posits that *your higher self is the driver of the car of your life*, and *you* as this specific human consciousness, *are the passenger.* You are not meant to be the one stressing about choices and directions, rather you are meant to relax and take in the view.

In theory, your higher self has already preselected your life trajectory and what will happen, and now you, in your human form, get to experience the roller coaster of living it. Instead of constantly stressing about what turn is going to happen next, you are meant to rely on your deeper knowing and be guided in each present moment by it instead. To put it bluntly, fucking let go already, you are not in control anyway.

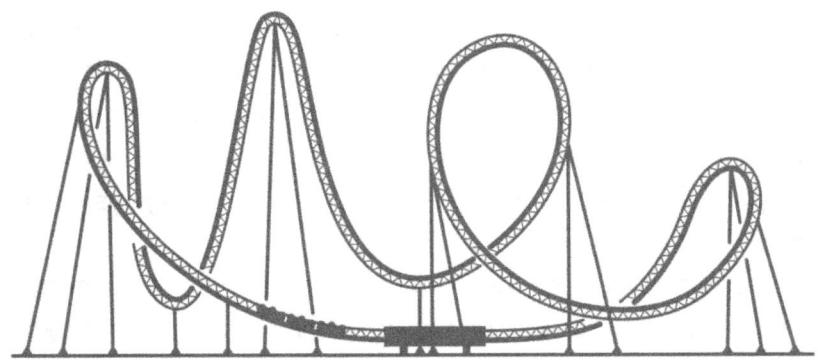

Now, living in this way does not somehow mean that pain will not happen. We are living a *human* life after all, so with that comes all the highs and lows, but it does mean that you can ride these highs and lows with less drama, trauma, and suffering.

Instead of being a boat tossed and thrashed by the unexpectedness of life, you become like a dolphin, sensing and adjusting to whatever state the ocean is in that day. Moreover, you gain a greater perspective of viewing life through a lens of long-term healing and evolution rather than short-term *seeking pleasure and avoiding pain.*

When life is lived this way, everything becomes *good* in that everything is *experienced.* You no longer resist and fight against the *bad* because you trust that *all of it is here for a reason.* Instead of spending the majority of your life and energy resisting *what is,* you spend it discovering the heights and depths of how much you can feel and who you truly are. This belief releases immense power normally conscripted by fear, anxiety, and confusion back into the flow of letting life be *lived through you.*

Belief #3: We slow down to speed up

As our world has sped up, so too has the expectation that we should be able to *keep up.* Normal cycles and rhythms have been discarded with the advent of artificial lighting, cell phones, computers, and the ability to work anywhere and at any time. These can be gifts when used wisely, but without foresight, we can easily fall into a pattern of go, go, go while never pausing to question where we're going and if the price we're paying to get there is worth it. This is where your nervous system comes in.

Currently we experience massive overstimulation of our nervous systems by just about everything in our culture; from chemically altered and stimulating foods to dopamine-jacking TVs and screens, we are surrounded by stimuli. All of this can lead to deep dysregulation of our nervous systems creating an almost total disconnect from our true felt sense in our bodies and a perpetual state of living up in our minds.

Just like those *Twilight Zone* movies about mind control, many of us are living more like robotic zombies programmed by whatever comes across our screens than true living and breathing humans.

In addition, the answer is ironically to slowwwwww dowwwwwwn. Way Way Down.

Once we slow down, we can tap back into the true source of knowledge in our bodies: a source that defies logic or science and yet has the most accurate and perfect answers for leading you through your one exquisitely-tailored-just-for-you-life.

The paradox is that as you slow down in your everyday life, you speed up in the creation of your most *aligned life.* This is because you spend far less time and energy on paths and ideas that are not meant for you. Paths that are only being pursued by your ego because it is seeking some sense of control from your nervous system being so over-stimulated and dysregulated.

Note to self: Wanting to control is just an indicator of dysregulation. The answer is not to go out and GET SOME MORE CONTROL, but to regulate. We do this by dropping in, dropping down, slowing down, making contact with our bodies, breathing deep, and accessing the peace that is here in the present. No amount of external seeking will ever give you the peace that comes from learning how to slow down and allow your nervous system to downregulate.

It's tempting to grasp for control, trying to reign in every detail. Yet, the elusive peace we seek isn't found in tightening our grip on the world around us. Instead, it emerges from within, from surrendering to the currents of the present moment and discovering tranquility in the heart of the storm.

Some of the best ways to do this are through somatic practices in the body. Just a few of my favorites are meditation, breath work, fascia release, yoga, ecstatic dance, sound healing, cupping, and therapeutic massage. Experiment and find the practices that work best for you. Until you befriend your body and work with it from a state of regulation, you will forever be putting out fires while ignoring the true source of the flames.

Belief #4: Trauma is real, and it is healed in the body, not just the mind

Believing that life is a dream can alleviate pressure and confusion, but it does not change the fact that we experience a wide range of sensations and emotions in our physical bodies.

We may feel overwhelming grief at the death of a loved one, excruciating fear and anxiety over a job loss or financial struggles, searing anger and caustic hatred towards those who have hurt us or others, and infinite combinations of other feelings and scenarios. If you look deeply at just one human's life you will realize quickly that the breadth and depth of the human experience is truly staggering.

In my work, I have learned that relying solely on cognitive behavioral approaches to handle emotions and trauma is not enough. This approach can trap individuals in a mental prison where they understand their trauma intellectually but do not process it in their body. This can be a new kind of hell where you know intellectually that you *should be able to change* and yet are perpetually hijacked by your trauma/nervous system thus exacerbating feelings of self-hatred and being stuck. Only by combining intellectual teachings with somatic emotional processing can true reconnection and self-healing begin.

Thankfully, we are seeing growing emphasis in our culture on the importance of not just mind work but also bodywork as well. Therapies such as EMDR, sensorimotor psychotherapy, and brain spotting are gaining popularity, not to mention the incredible effects being found in research around the healing potentials of psychedelics, MDMA, and LSD.

This growing awareness points to the reality that trauma from our childhoods and our pasts cannot just be "gotten over" by shoving it down deep and never looking at it again. That shit will come out in all sorts of unconscious ways like the adult games we play of shaming, blaming, and judging ourselves that are really just childhood patterns of self-abandonment. If we're honest, many of us are just children walking around in adult bodies pretending like we know what we're doing while inwardly feeling crushing dread, terror, and overwhelm for most of our lives.

The answer begins with acknowledging you have trauma and that your trauma is real. From there you get to embark on a journey to heal your relationship with your inner child. This work can be facilitated in all kinds of ways and everyone's journey is different but what is most important is feeling into where your next step is and taking it.

At various times mine and my client's *next steps* have looked like taking a pottery class, going back to school, working with a coach, reading a book on NPD disorder, or laying in a hammock for five minutes each day. The *what* is not nearly as important as the *why* and your why will sound something like, "Because it just feels right. Because something inside me just wants to." You are looking for a sensation in your gut similar to how it feels just before you go down a roller coaster or when your heart feels like it skips a tiny beat. It may feel simultaneously exciting and terrifying. If so, good. You are getting it.

Once you have even the tiniest of these impressions, follow it, no matter how small. Each one will show you a way to heal your trauma and reconnect with the inner parts you disowned to survive and are now ready to reclaim.

In this reclamation, you experience wholeness again and the energy that was being used to suppress your painful parts is now free to help you create a truly soul-led life.

Belief #5: Every time you heal for yourself, you heal for the collective

This work can be challenging. At times, you may feel like you are carrying the karmic burdens of thousands as you bravely cut a new path through the untamed wilderness of your own pain and suffering. In those moments, it can mean everything to know that what you are doing matters not just to you, but also to the entire human collective.

In reading the words of those who have attained deep levels of peace in this world, a powerful theme emerged; we are all part of *The One*. Like fingers on a hand, we look around and see separation, but the reality is that we are all part of the same organism, an interconnected and energetic source that runs through each one of us in this world.

For those who have done psychedelics or had moments of powerful enlightenment, you know that this *One* holds deep and unfathomable realms of creation, humanity, and worlds without end. Some will call this Source, some God, and some The Universe among many other hundreds of names. It is less about *what* it is called and more about how it makes you *feel* when you connect to it.

Believing in this source allows us to tap into something much greater than ourselves. Knowing this greater scale exists helps us flow between the microcosms of our own deeply important personal lives and the macrocosm of the evolution of our species as a whole. Each of our lives plays a part in how that evolution unfolds.

In my journey, I have faced emotional moments that felt bigger than I did. Moments where I felt like I was processing not just my fear and grief but also that of my ancestral mothers and grandmothers who had grown up in environments less supportive of women's freedom. I believe this weight is the karmic remains of the *One* "growing up."

Just like each of us passes through developmental stages of life, I believe the One is also going through its own stages. Throughout history, we have seen a "two-steps forward, one-step back" approach to evolution, but always with an overarching trend towards more consciousness.

Although we still see war, poverty, neglect, abuse, and corruption, we also see a growing consciousness that abolishes slavery, abhors genocide and war, and expects equality for all regardless of gender, race, or sexual orientation. The collective consciousness (The One) is learning *who it wants to be* through generations of humans living out their lives and choosing *who they want to be*. With each life lived, we step forward even further into the light or retreat backward into the dark.

This is why those of us called to lives of transmutation are so important. In the span of just one lifetime, we can change these generational karmic patterns and stop them from repeating. We can end cycles of abuse, transform trauma, and transmute ignorance into knowledge and pain into self-trust. You do not have to go out and *change the world* to change the world. You can heal within, and the world changes from there.

Final thoughts

No one knows what we're doing here. Yes, I have shared ideas with you and there are thousands more out there; just walk into any church on a Sunday or pick up a book from the self-help section. That is exactly why the most important thing you can do is learn how to recognize and follow your OWN soul-led calls. No one outside of you has your answers.

When we do not follow our soul calls, we end up living lives that look reasonable on the outside but feel unfulfilling on the inside. Most of us hide daily from this truth by spending our whole lives caught up in the perpetual seeking of external control. In this way, we waste our *one precious life* on a hamster wheel of distraction, addiction, and disconnection. Huge amounts of powerful unused human potential are trapped right now in individuals who stay in marriages, careers, and locations that do not feed their souls but feel eerily comfortable in a static generational way.

If more people choose to live soul-led lives, we could unlock an unfathomable amount of energy and talents, shifting our collective reality and changing our species' trajectory in just one to two generations.

To do so, start with one small soul-led shift from the list at the end of the chapter.

It is only by taking the road less traveled that we can bring about real change and pave the way for a better future. Whatever your next step may be, take it with courage and conviction. Let it be a declaration to yourself that you are ready to live a life led by your soul and that you are committed to expanding human potential.

Remember that every step forward is a testament to your resilience and determination. Every step is an opportunity to embrace the unknown with open arms, for it is in the depths of uncertainty that our true strength is revealed. As we bravely face our fears and step out into the unfamiliar, what we find is the boldness and resilience we've been hungering for our whole lives.

I promise that you will draw unparalleled strength from the challenges you face. Know that they are the very experiences shaping you into the person you are meant to become.

Trust that it is safe to embrace uncertainty and allow for all the human messiness of your journey ahead. It is only in stepping out into the dark of the unknown to follow our soul calls that we uncover the true extent of our personal power and potential.

Be willing to push the edges; the possibilities are endless, and the future is bright for those who dare to dream big and take soul-led action.

Key takeaways to implement

Practices for a soul-led life: start with one small soul-led shift. It could be testing out one of the beliefs I have shared, trying something that popped into your head just now, or something from the list below:

* Start reading that book that's been calling to you.

* Reach out to that person that's been on your mind lately.

* Say no to that thing you don't want to do but have been making yourself do to keep others happy.

* Share one of your deepest most vulnerable, and yet unfulfilled, hopes for your life with a friend.

* Give yourself five minutes to breathe deeply while placing your hands on your heart. Notice any sensations that arise in your body. Allow them with love.

* Acknowledge aloud to yourself any person, habit, substance, or activity that you are currently engaging with that does not support you in living a soul-led life.

* Start working with that coach or mentor who inspires you and lights you up whenever you hear them speak.

* Notice what you feel excited about and go do one thing this week related to that.

About the author

Britta Jo is a fiercely compassionate coach, podcast host, and founder of *The Stay or Go Community*—a radically supportive space for women standing at the crossroads of their marriage and identity. After unraveling her own life—leaving Mormonism, identifying narcissistic abuse in her family and marriage, and shedding layers of patriarchal smallness—she rebuilt everything from the inside out, guided by radical intuition and soul trust. Now, through her community, podcast, and private coaching she helps women get unstuck and move forward to create juicy, full lives that reflect the wild, wise creatures they've always been. Known for her raw realness and unshakable devotion to women's freedom, she's on the cutting edge of how we talk about considering divorce—not as failure, but as a portal to power, aliveness, and living a soul-led life.

stayorgocoaching.com

Patricia's decades of firsthand experience with the sanitization of death leaves a profound impression. She offers wisdom for navigating the challenging terrain of end-of-life, enhancing both the dying process for families and our daily living through embracing mortality as part of life.

Her message about honoring death as part of life is one our culture desperately needs.

— *Book momma Chandra*

18

The Sacred Exit: The Journey of Sacred Passages

Patricia Moir Pollman RN NC-BC

Death is a condition common to all matter.

A recent survey asked Americans what their greatest fear is; their number one response is death. Fears were of physical pain and suffering, loss, grief, and isolation. From being a registered nurse for many years, I have learned much from people in their dying process. Now, as a life and death coaching companion — I would like to share with you, gentle readers, what *Death* has taught me.

Much of the fear of death arises from how medical care has been delivered in the past 40 to 50 years. With the advances in medicine, and technology, great progress has been made in averting grave health crises like heart attack and stroke. However, we have come to believe there is a cure for everything. In the past, loved ones and family members were present as caregivers during serious, and end of life illness. Families were present the changing advances; they witnessed the decreasing quality of life each day. They kept vigil.

But as medical care became more advanced, the role of family members as caregivers diminished, the deep familiarity of death was lifted, and the fear of it grew. With the advent of high-tech medicine, hospitals became the primary site of care, and the rituals of dying at home were replaced with the sterile and impersonal environment of the hospital. The dying process became more hidden, more sanitized, more distant, unknown, and scarier.

If you are facing death yourself or have a loved one facing death: I write to both of you to unveil the mystery, relieve fear, and to open the needed conversation and the unknown choices around the death process.

Modern death

I have watched many people who are left to face their own mortality without the benefit of a shared experience with loved ones. They are forced to confront their own fears and anxieties in isolation, without the comfort and support of those who hold the wisdom of death. Death has become a solo journey, devoid of the warmth, love, and acceptance that comes from being surrounded by those who care.

The hospitals that most are admitted to now deliver life-lengthening interventions, without a conversation about their options including quality versus quantity of life. Many die with families excluded from the all-important process of caring for their loved one — creating crippling grief that is difficult to recover from.

In order to heal modern death, I offer a vision of re-imagining death by returning to caring for the whole person, a model of providing information for informed choices, and a relationship-centered approach for the whole family. Here, the divinity and sanctity of life and death can be restored with dignity and grace, in alignment with the dying person's values along with the well-being of the family left behind.

Your invite to re-imagine death

I invite you to think of death, not as an enemy to be feared, but as your greatest teacher revealing what is most important to you in your life as you live.

Death and life are forever intertwined and cannot be separated from one another. Death and life are two sides of the same coin, inseparable like the threads of a tapestry. They are not opposing forces, but complementary aspects of the human experience. One cannot exist without the other, and yet, we often try to separate them, to treat them as distinct entities.

The current trend with death is both to attempt to prolong life and to defy death. Developing medicines, technologies, and therapies attempting to extend days as well as to keep bodies and minds functioning. And yet, in the zeal to prolong life, the reality that death is an integral part of the human experience is repressed.

What if rather than repressing death's inevitability, you instead invite death into your life as an aspect of your life? This will allow your humanity to be enriched, so that when the last breath is drawn it will be free of regret; instead, you will be filled with grace, peace, and dignity. Living and dying with the ability to express and embrace your full human potential.

As a human being, you are by nature whole: body, mind, heart, and soul. A fully alive life, and death, is experienced when all aspects are coherent and aligned.

Living in the fear of your death, paralyzes your ability to explore, expand, make choices, and experience the depths of being — that embracing death offers. By embracing death, you can choose how, where, and with whom you make your death-journey — affecting your quality of life while dying.

Living while dying is a magnificent, triumphant
expression of being human.

Recognize and allow death into your life as an integral aspect of being human. Take death's hand, walk with it, and you will learn how you want to live, to be remembered, and loved.

Perhaps death's shadow will illuminate each second of your life, and you will come to know the silver linings. Come to know it as a vital, purposeful stage of human development, just like birth, childhood, adolescence, adulthood, and elderhood. Each stage is a thread that weaves the rich tapestry of your life. At the end of your life, this tapestry will fill you with memories, joy, and the knowingness of a life well lived.

When at death's door

Consider examining holistic care for both your loved one at death's door and the those who love and care for the dying. Become informed, do research, learn about your options.

In service to humanity, I begin the conversation of how these needs could be met, starting with the dying and their loved ones to be the ones in control. Second, accepting death as a natural process and a part of life. Then third, exploring the possibilities of death's transition.

No *one way* to die

There is no single right or wrong way to offer and provide care at this stage of life. You get to choose.

People continue to live even while in the process of dying.

Addressing pain and symptoms well frees the individual to have the energy to be curious about what they want — today, tomorrow, and at the last moment. End of life practitioners are skilled at effective management of pain and symptoms to relieve unnecessary suffering.

For the dying

- Imagine spreading a banquet table rich with your memories, filled with the awareness of the human you have been and are also becoming in the same moment.

- Imagine displaying a feast of your human expression unafraid to be known; knowledge and memories of you that can be kept forever in the heart of all who knew and loved you.

- Consider leading your journey into the unknown as a human with the courage to express yourself vulnerably and authentically; know it is possible for you to be an inspiration for those who remain.

- Let go of guilt, fear, and helplessness.

- Fill yourself with precious memories; know you have air beneath your angel wings.

- Consider allowing a loved one to guide you through the below *Manner of Death's Inquiry.*

In these depths of our being we may discover our highest and most creative potential. Within this potential, we are again sacred beings.

Manner of Death's Inquiry: Support guide for end of life

Once the physical aspects are well managed, encourage the dying to go through this inquiry and talk about who they are, what is important to them, and who they want to be around them at this time.

Support guide questions for meaningful conversations at the end of life

1. Understanding wishes and beliefs

- How do you see your illness progressing, and are there things you'd like to know or prepare for?

- How would you like to be remembered?

- What are your wishes for how your remains should be cared for?

- What do you believe about death and what comes after it?
- Are there any religious or spiritual beliefs that bring you comfort as you face this time?

2. Healing and forgiveness

- Are there relationships you feel need healing or people you would like to reconnect with?
- Is there anyone you need to forgive or anyone from whom you'd like to seek forgiveness?
- How do you feel about the idea of healing — not just of the body, but of the heart and mind?

3. Exploring thoughts and feelings

- What fears or worries are present for you right now?
- What feelings or thoughts would you like to share?
- How can I create a space for you where you feel safe to express yourself without judgment?

4. Presence and connection

- Who do you want to be with you during this time?
- How can I or others best support you in feeling dignity and grace as you near the end of your life?
- What does being fully present with yourself look like?

5. Honoring final wishes

- Are there any specific wishes or last desires you want us to honor?
- What does a peaceful environment look like for you? How can we create that for you?

6. Love and legacy

- How can we bring love and peace into this space for you?

- Are there memories, stories, or wisdom you'd like to share with your loved ones?

7. Empowering care

- How can we, as those who love you, care for you in a way that supports your desires and needs?

- What is the most important thing we can do to show our love for you right now?

These open-ended questions can foster deeper understanding, connection, and peace during this profound time, helping the dying person feel seen, heard, and cherished. Encourage them to guide the pace and direction of these conversations, creating a space for honesty, vulnerability, and love.

Spiritual integrity is to face the unknown together.

If spiritual integrity resonates with you, know the above exercise is one you and your loved ones can use to create an experience of spiritual integrity.

In this Manner of Inquiry above, fear has been allayed, the mind truthfully informed, the body cared for with dignity, and desires respected — here, the strength, wisdom, and power of human potential is realized — the spirit has spoken and is given freedom. All involved are honoring this dear life and creating a celebration of a life lived well and a death experienced with dignity, peace, harmony, and grace — the dying is able to soar free of human constraints.

The vigil: For loved ones supporting the dying

Before death
As death draws nearer, the skin changes color and becomes cooler to the touch. The breath becomes more ragged.

- Tell stories.

- Share memories and photographs.

- Let the family pet lay together with the patient.

- Encourage visitation from those who knew and loved this wonderful human.

- Touch gently.

- Speak softly into their ear of your loving memories — give thanks for what they have meant in your life.

The moment of death
The threshold between life and eternity, a boundary where the breath of existence falters, and the veil of mortality parts. In this stillness, the eyes remain closed, as if the soul has finally found rest. The silence is palpable, a hush that wraps around the heart like a gentle shroud.

- It is time to say your farewells.

- Know you do not need to hasten to call the funeral home.

- Take all the time you need and want.

- Bathing, anointing, and dressing the loved one for their departure from this life journey can serve as the last token of your respect and esteem. This could be your last loving act which will remain in your heart for days to come.

Embrace the satisfaction you may feel, knowing that your loved ones are in a better place, and you gave them the last goodbye — this will be your silver lining.

Losing a relative, family member, spouse or a friend is heart-wrenching. Believing that you may meet them one day will give you courage and hope to keep living.

Burial choices after death

Burial and cremation are options that are becoming fewer. The land cannot continue to support our dead burials, and cremation is being recognized as toxic to the air and the soil on our small blue planet Earth.

New choices arise. Green burial choices grow. Becoming aware of current choices allows you to care for your loved departed and Earth.

It has been my sincere honor to share what the dying have taught me about this vital stage of life.

A poem of comfort

Why?
That is what we ask.
The truth is, we may never be able to know for sure why.
However, we do know that there is no single
"Should have done,"
Or "Would have done,"
Or "Did," or "Didn't do"
That would have changed the Why.
All that love could do was done.

— Unknown author

I am grateful for the opportunity to serve. By visioning a potential re-imagining of death, one that you can embrace to authentically enrich each day of your life.

What you may experience as expanded consciousness during death and dying need not be reserved for this stage of life but instead, become a portal for curiosity and wonder about the potential of your human life.

May many blessings be with you

May the gentle breeze of hope blow upon you,
Bringing calm to your soul and peace to your mind.
May the warmth of kindness shine upon your face,
Guiding you through life's challenges and difficulties.

May the blessings of the heavens be yours to claim,
Gratitude for every breath, every moment, every name.
May the light of hope illuminate your path,
Leading you to triumph over every obstacle.

May your heart be filled with joy and your spirit be free,
From the chains of worry and the weight of anxiety.
May your mind be at peace, like a still pond on a summer's day,
Reflecting the beauty and wonder of life's journey.

May many blessings be with you, dear one,
Guiding, protecting, and keeping you safe until you are home.
May you walk in faith, knowing that you are not alone,
Surrounded by the love and care of those who have gone
before.

May this blessing be a source of comfort and strength to you,
A reminder that you are loved, cherished, and forever true.
May it bring you peace, hope, and joy, in every moment and
every day,
And may you always know that many blessings are on their way.

— Unknown author

With that note, thank you, dear and gentle reader, for spending your precious time with me. Together in realizing your highest human potential for the greatest good of all.

Key takeaways to implement

* For loved ones and the dying — ask yourself: What must I do to-day, to be at peace with myself, so that I may live this ever-present moment and become able to die in grace, with dignity, without regret, or fear, aware and self-realized?

* For the dying — decide on: What do you want your tombstone to say about who you were, besides dates and names?

* Reclaim the interconnectedness of life, death, and all sentient beings.

* Pass this chapter to someone who is involved with the dying process.

* Come back to the chapter and use it when you need it to care for a loved one in their dying process, or your own.

About the author

Patricia was born in Aberdeen, Scotland and immigrated to America in 1968, arriving in Reno in 1971, where she has served her community as an RN in Reno hospitals, across many specialty areas, including: hospice, palliative care, end of life care, and elder advocacy.

She has completed many studies including: end of life practitioner for re-imagining the end of life.

It is Patricia's passion to serve and support her clients in clarifying and envisioning their goals and purpose and in achieving their highest good and wellbeing through all of life transitions and stages: in health, wellness, illness, and in dying — by creating a sacred, safe, and healing space where clients can find and express their unique human potential.

Consider allowing me to walk with you, as a companion and guide, as a witness to your strength, courage and life experience, your inner knowing, vulnerability and pain you have overcome, and perhaps recover, the parts of you that may have become separated or lost upon the journey we call life. To call back that eternal you, that speaks throughout the ages of the ever present you.

pp93571@aol.com

Epilogue
Life Design 101

Cut out everything unnecessary and extra.
Focus on what is important.
Nourish your Self and what you love.
Review, reflect, rewrite.

Change it up.
Stop. Slow down. Sprint. Fly.

Wondering where time goes?
Catch your thoughts.
Harness your life force.

Get angry with the world.
Fight for something better.
Relax. Accept.
Lower expectations.
Keep fighting the good fight.

Lean into differences.
Rock the boat.
Embrace challenge.

End your day satisfied.
Wake grateful.
Another day on this side of the earth.
Another breath to breathe.
Another moment to be.
Before we rejoin the stardust.

Time does not exist.
We construct measurements
in order to create order.
Seek your balance
between order and chaos.
You are unique and need your own specific number.

Do not follow the herd.
You are more than a number.
You are more than a soldier.
Be the version of you that is alive and thriving.

Question everything.
Buy less.
Give more.
Sing and dance daily.

Get naked.
Undress your heart.
Show your vulnerable side.
Allow yourself to bleed tears.
This will clean you out.

Strength is the courage to be vulnerable.
Express your love.
Love is the true richness of life.

Make enough money,
but know that making money
will not give you happiness.
Happiness is something
that comes from the inside.
If you are working your life away
for the "forever away future"
you will miss living it.
There are many chances in life,
but most only come around once.
Know your Self,
so that when your chance comes you know it is yours.

Talk to yourself,
go on walks,
ask deep questions.
Discover what makes you tick
and what makes you sick.

Be ruthless in your boundaries,
you owe very few people,
do not give away your life-force,
they may not give it back.

Empower those around you.
Let go of dying friendships
before you are pulled down
an unwanted rabbit hole.
Always choose love,
it is always an option.

Imagine your life.
Build it. Breathe it.
Work your ass off through the discomfort of change.
Pause, reflect, rest.
Tune back in. Take off.

Find home within your bones.
Reside within your heart.
Take up space.
Make your Self bigger.
Expand your lungs.
Breathe fire into your eyes.

Love yourself as you want others to love you.
You are your first human to attend to.

When you come to your lover
with your own needs met,
then you have the opportunity for True Love.

Tune into those around you.
Learn the innate life changing power of empathy.
Put yourself in other's shoes.

Within your head and heart, walk in their footsteps.
Understand their position.
Imagine their pain.
Love them not in spite of their pain
but because of it.

Rock your life like you have only one.
Because the odds are that you do have only this one life.
This crazy amazing evolutionary phenomena is You
and everything you see and do not see around you.

What is the point of life?
To grow. To love, and to embrace life's duality.

You will be on your deathbed,
judging your life.
You will know if you cheated your Self,
you *know* if you are allowing your Self to miss.

Catch yourself in the moment.
Be the person you are proud of.

Self-care. Express. Breathe. Eat. Connect. Reflect.
All lead you to
  – be true to your Self.

—Chandra Zas

The words you just read in "Life Design 101" are invitations to step into the fullest expression of who you want to be. They speak to the part of you that knows there is more to life than what you have been settling for, the part that is ready to start celebrating the potential within you.

This isn't the end — it's another step on the path, another piece of the puzzle of your potential. Scan the QR code or visit handbookforhumanpotential.com to discover more about each author, connect with us on social media, and deepen your journey. If this book has sparked something in you, share it — gift it to fellow growth seekers and keep the ripple of transformation going. The more we invest in our own growth, the more we expand what's possible for all of us.

www.handbookforhumanpotential.com

Acknowledgments

This book represents a collaborative effort that stretched me in ways I never imagined. There were moments I considered giving up: I sat with that possibility and chose to keep going. What emerged from that choice was something far greater than I could have created alone. This book demanded so much more than I anticipated, and I am deeply grateful it is finally ready to reach you.

Thank you to every contributing author for your exceptional chapters and your thoughtful feedback throughout every stage of this process. Most importantly, thank you for the grace and patience you offered when this journey took longer than expected. Your understanding and grace made all the difference.

I want to give special recognition to Heidi Jo Wayco. Thank you for teaching me how to edit, how to navigate Word, and for the many heartfelt conversations that kept me going when I needed them most. Thank you for the genuine friendship we created through this endeavor. And thank you, Jim, for the introduction that started it all.

Thank you, Mac, for introducing me to Jeffrey Kripal. Jeffrey, thank you for the beautiful foreword and for connecting me with Sharon. Sharon, your professionalism and exceptional formatting skills are remarkable, my deepest gratitude.

✳

Thank you to my dedicated proofreaders. To Stav and Burton, your scientific expertise and honest feedback when you found the opening chapter challenging led me to reorganize the entire structure and create a new opening chapter. That insight was invaluable. To Elizabeth, your meticulous attention to detail caught so many errors that will make a significant difference in the final product. To my mom, Sherry, thank you for helping me navigate big-picture decisions, for your financial support, and for being my most enthusiastic cheerleader.

✳

Seth, thank you for guiding me through the world of publicity. Let's get this book into many hands, hearts, and minds.

✳

I would also like to extend a special thank you to Michael Murphy, whose creation of the Esalen Institute served as a vital incubator for the human potential movement. My five years of living, working, and studying at Esalen profoundly influenced my personal journey and provided the initial spark for this book. It was there that I befriended Mac Murphy, who, nearly twenty years later, was one of the first people I turned to when deciding to create this handbook. Their combined influence represents a remarkable, multigenerational legacy. Where Michael provided the visionary framework for the movement, Mac embodies its principles through hands-on, somatic practices. Their work demonstrates a beautiful evolution of human potential, from its intellectual origins to the deeply embodied and ecological approaches we explore today.

✳

Finally, thank you to you, the readers, for investing in this book and in your own personal growth. This book was created for you, as a tool for developing your potential. My hope is that together, we can help raise our collective potential. Please share this book, pass it along, give it as a gift, and let's create a collective consciousness shift, one reader at a time.